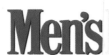

BEST

THE 15 BEST
EXERCISES

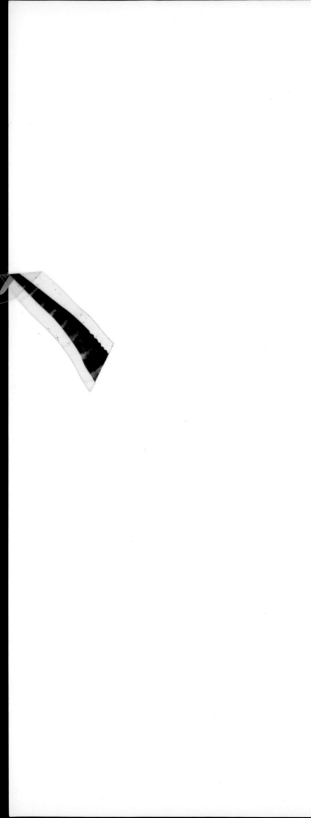

Men's Health® BEST

THE 15 BEST EXERCISES

SECRETS FROM *MEN'S HEALTH* MAGAZINE

Edited by **Joe Kita**, *Men's Health* magazine

RODALE®

This edition first published in 2005 by
Rodale International Ltd
7–10 Chandos Street
London
W1G 9AD
www.rodalebooks.co.uk

"Men's Health®" is a registered trademark of Rodale Inc.

Cover photograph by Andrew Southam; back cover photograph by Getty Images.

Interior Photographs
Brand X Pictures: 18, 20, 25; Comstock: 76, 78; Corbis: 13, 22, 74; Digital Vision: 6, 8, 82, 85, 90; Dave Krieger: 12, 14; Michael Mazzeo: 11, 26–70, 72–73, 79–81, 87–89; Sean Murphy: 71; Tom Rafalovich: 16; Think Stock: image in running head, 86; Miranda Penn Turrin: 9.

Printed and bound in China.
3 5 7 9 8 6 4 2

A CIP catalogue record for this book is available from the British Library.

ISBN 1-4050-7763-8

Notice
The information in this book is meant to supplement, not replace, proper exercise training. All forms of exercise pose some inherent risks. The editors and publisher advise readers to take full responsibility for their safety and know their limits. Before practising the exercises in this book, be sure that your equipment is well maintained, and do not take risks beyond your level of experience, aptitude, training and fitness.

The exercise and dietary programmes in this book are not intended as a substitute for any exercise routine or dietary regime that may have been prescribed by your doctor. As with all exercise and dietary programmes, you should get your doctor's approval before beginning.

Visit us on the Web at *www.menshealth.co.uk*

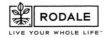

LIVE YOUR WHOLE LIFE™

We inspire and enable people to improve their lives and the world around them

CONTENTS

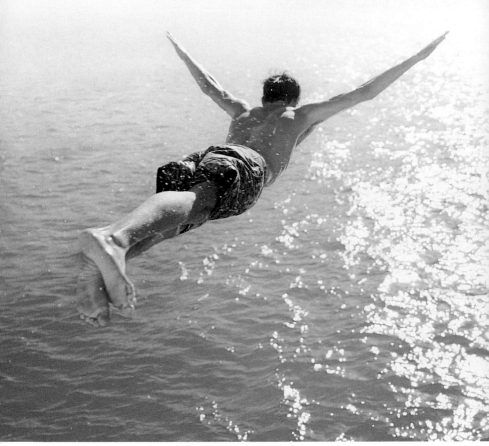

The 15 exercises in this book work every major muscle group. What are you waiting for? Dive in.

INTRODUCTION

Welcome to *Men's Health's Best: The 15 Best Exercises*. This book is intended for novices, seasoned fitness veterans, the curious and the sceptical. As you hold this book you may be thinking: why are these the 15 best exercises? And what exactly do they mean by 'best', anyway?

In evaluating countless (okay, hundreds) of candidates for this list, it became clear that 'best' need not include anything particularly complex or difficult in order to make a difference in the building of strength, power and fitness. Spelling things out for the purposes of this book, 'best' means fundamental and 'exercise' means a strength-training exercise as opposed to aerobic exercise. That's why, when you're flicking through the pages, you won't find discussions of running, walking, swimming or skipping. (All of these are aerobic activities that raise your heart rate and burn calories without necessarily building muscle mass.) You will find exercises that build muscle through weight resistance, whether the weight is external (as in a dumbbell) or your own body weight (as in a Press-up or Pull-up).

These 15 exercises work all the major muscle groups: shoulders, chest, arms, upper and lower back, and legs. They represent a variety of methods: bench exercises, floor exercises, hanging exercises, those that involve pushing weights, exercises that involve pulling weights and so on. The editors of *Men's Health* arrived at this list by interviewing exercise physiologists, fitness experts, personal trainers and athletes. Their knowledge is now your knowledge.

Part I (page 9) is divided into three sections. In 'Meet Your 15 Best Exercises' you'll learn the basics about the exercises and the muscle groups they work. In 'Diet and Nutrition' you'll get the lowdown on the latest research to get you started

on a balanced approach to gaining muscle and losing fat. Whether you're ravenous at the end of your first workout, wondering how to get yourself revved up for morning exercise or out of steam before you've completed a circuit, this section has answers, and a meal plan, for you. In 'Stretch, Then Stretch Some More' you'll find a five-page flexibility

THE 15 BEST EXERCISES

Here's a preview of the 15 exercises selected by the editors of *Men's Health*. Feel free to flick straight to your favourite. If you're curious about the runners-up, check out 'Just a Few More' on page 65.

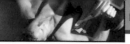

primer to make sure you approach each of the exercises with warm, supple muscles.

Part II (page 31) takes you through all of the 15 best exercises step-by-step, with a wide range of variations for when you've mastered the basics. Part III (page 71) answers the question, 'How do I put all 15 exercises to use in a workout?'

It features three full exercise programmes and four miniworkout circuits that address all the major muscle groups and are designed to push the essential 15 to their limits (and yours).

So we've simplified the world of muscle building and fitness for you. Now is your chance to take advantage of what's here.

The more time you spend working out indoors, the more improvement you'll see in what you can do in the great outdoors.

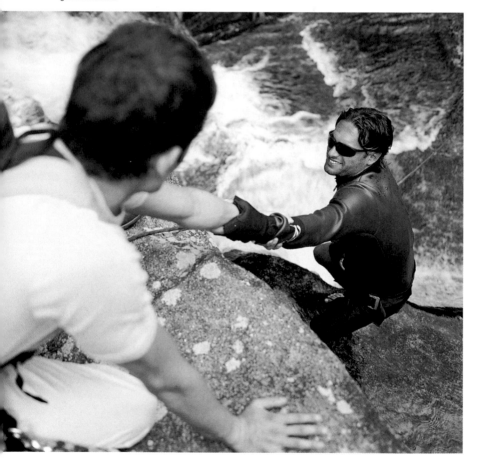

PART I:
Total Body Basics

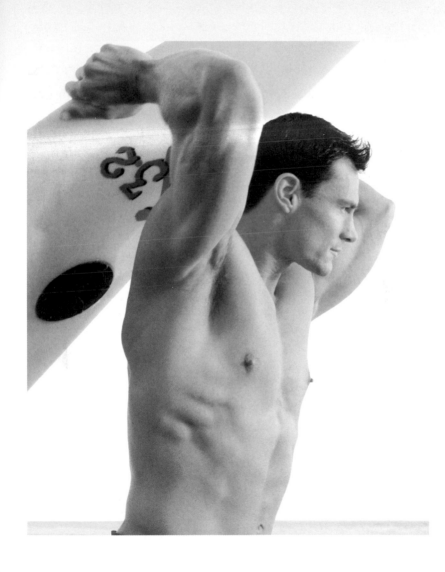

Meet Your 15 Best Exercises

These are the fundamentals – the ingredients that go into the ultimate recipe, your workout. Take a look at the major muscle groups (shown at right) that receive a workout from these workhorses. Then watch these muscles develop as you learn proper form and the rhythm of each exercise, and start to use the multitude of variations you'll find in Part II (page 31). On the bench, chair or floor, hanging from your arms or standing before what was once an impossible barbell load, these 15 exercises are where it all starts.

Bench Press

An essential part of any strength-training programme, the Bench Press (also known as a chest press) works the pectoralis major, the fan-shaped muscles that cover the upper chest. (The pecs are the thick muscles that move your upper arms in towards your chest when you push your arms out in front of you.) This exercise also works the anterior deltoids (at the top of the shoulder, responsible for raising your arms in front of you) and the triceps (at the back of the upper arm, a three-part muscle that straightens your arm). The Bench Press is the benchmark move for weight trainers, many of whom often boil an entire workout down to the question, 'How much can you bench?'

TEST THE BENCH

Before you start, make sure the bench is going to be a reliable workout partner: press your thumb into the bench before lifting. If you can feel the wood, find another bench. Hard benches can cause T4 syndrome – a misalignment of your thoracic (upper) spine that affects the nerve function of your arms, weakening them.

Press-up

There's a reason your high school gym teacher had you doing endless Press-ups all those years ago. It's the

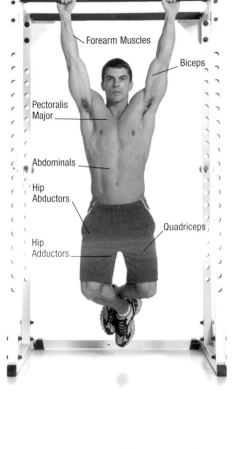

Forearm Muscles

Biceps

Pectoralis Major

Abdominals

Hip Abductors

Quadriceps

Hip Adductors

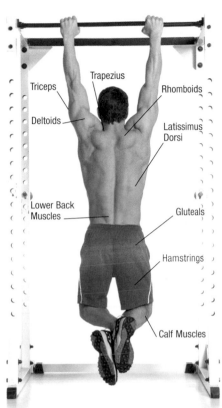

Trapezius

Triceps

Rhomboids

Deltoids

Latissimus Dorsi

Lower Back Muscles

Gluteals

Hamstrings

Calf Muscles

same reason you'll see professional athletes and soldiers performing this move wherever they can. The Press-up works the same set of muscles as the Bench Press (the pectoralis major, anterior deltoids and triceps), but it requires no bench and no weights. Think of a Press-up as a Bench Press turned upside down, where your body weight substitutes for a barbell and gravity provides the resistance. The only requirement for

OVERCOME INJURIES, BUILD BIG ARMS

If you have injured your right arm, don't stop exercising your left arm. Research has found that people who train only one arm for two weeks actually manage to increase arm strength in their non-exercising arm by up to 10 per cent. The reason? Exercising one arm stimulates the muscle nerve fibres in the opposite arm.

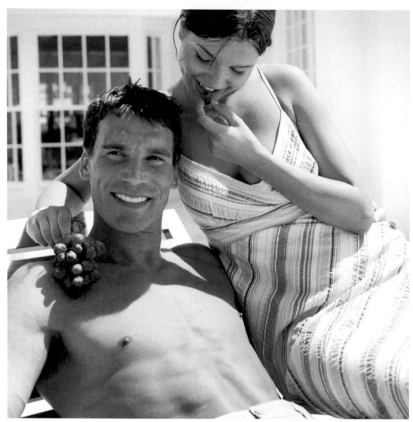

Eating right and maintaining a healthy lifestyle can help you to make lots of new friends.

a press-up is the will to face your own limitations and the desire to push yourself past them.

Curl

You've probably known this move since you were a kid, when you thought strength was synonymous with big biceps (the two-part muscles at the front of the upper arm responsible for bending it). Although the biceps are the major focus of this exercise, the Curl also works the brachioradialis (the muscle at the top of the forearm). What's so great about having fully developed biceps? Strong biceps aid in such a wide variety of exercises that it's impossible to have a well-developed back, abdomen or chest without them.

Shoulder Press

This exercise is an integral part of any upper-body workout. The Shoulder Press targets the triceps, deltoids and especially the middle delts (which are responsible for raising your arms to the side and above your head). The Shoulder Press is a great antidote to the common problem of overworking the biceps and anterior delts through the Bench Press and Press-up. By targeting the lesser-worked middle delts and triceps, the Shoulder Press may have single-handedly inspired the adage 'No pain, no gain'. Please note that the military press is one of many variations of the Shoulder Press. The classic military press is done standing, with a barbell, and you need to work extra hard to make sure you keep the back's natural alignment and don't bend.

Dip

This challenging exercise works three major muscle groups at the same time: the deltoids, the pectoralis major and the triceps. Because of this, it's often at the heart of many workout programmes. Dips can be tough, because you can't use lighter weights while you are learning proper form. But there is help out there to master the Dip, in the form of an assisted Dip machine, which enables you to learn the move without having to bear your entire body weight. If your gym doesn't have one, you might like to point out the machine's benefits and politely suggest they get one!

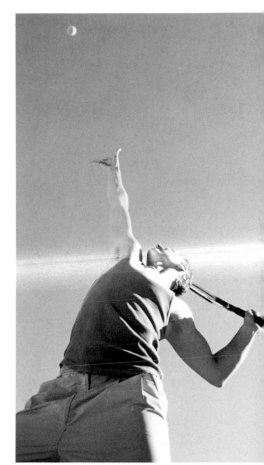

Improvements in conditioning and stamina will pay dividends for you on the tennis court – especially in the fifth set, when your opponent may be wearing down.

DOUBLE DIP BENEFITS

Do dips with your elbows in and your body straight to work your triceps. You can lean forwards and flare your elbows out to focus on your chest.

Row

There are many varieties of Row exercises, but they all generally target the same group of upper-body muscles. The first group is the latissimus dorsi, the big back muscles that give you that coveted V-shape and that pull your upper arms towards you as you do the rowing movement. The next group is the trapezius, the diamond-shaped muscle in your upper back, neck and shoulders that is responsible for moving your shoulder blades up and down, as in a shoulder shrug, or pushed back, as when a soldier snaps to attention. Don't forget about the posterior deltoids, which are responsible for pulling your arms backwards. And finally, there's the integral biceps muscle – although the Row is actually much more targeted to the back muscles that work *with* the biceps to move your arms forwards and backwards.

Pull-ups and Hanging Knee Raises are among the most difficult exercises, but they are among the best ways to strengthen your back, not to mention your arms.

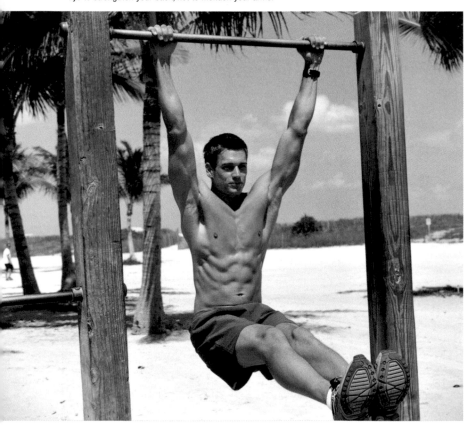

Pull-up

Like the Dip, the Pull-up may seem exceptionally challenging at first, and some guys need an assisted Pull-up machine (or an ordinary chair) to practise good form and get the hang of it. Pull-ups work the muscles of the back, especially the trapezius, the rhomboids (a pair of muscles in the upper back under the trapezius), the posterior deltoids, the latissimus dorsi (which move the arms away from the body), the teres major (much smaller muscles that assist the latissimus dorsi) and the biceps. The biceps will get more of a workout in a Pull-up in which the palms face the body than one that uses an overhand grip. The overhand grip puts more of an emphasis on the back muscles.

Fly

Shortened from 'butterfly', which refers to this exercise's wing-like movement, the Fly has the distinction of isolating the pectoralis major – unlike the Bench Press, Press-up and Dip, which also work the deltoids and triceps. It's sink or swim for the pecs, which inspires many novices to arch their backs and pump their legs in a vain (and often undignified) attempt to assist their struggling chest muscles in this crucial move.

Back Extension

This exercise is crucial in building lower-back strength, ensuring good posture and helping ward off the lower-back pain that so many people experience. It targets the erector spinae – the large muscles that run along the sides of the lower back and help to support the spine.

Hanging Knee Raise

Like the Dip and the Pull-up, the Hanging Knee Raise uses your body weight for resistance. It targets the obliques, a pair of muscles that run diagonally along the sides of your torso and are responsible for its ability to flex. It also works the lower portion of the rectus abdominis, the large muscle that flexes the torso forwards and backwards. This muscle is

POSITIVE THINKING

Seeing improvement guarantees more improvement. Try keeping a training diary and record weight lifted, sets and repetitions for each exercise. Also record your body weight and measurements. Doing so will not only enable you to track your progress, but it will also keep you excited about your training, which lays the groundwork for more perfect workouts.

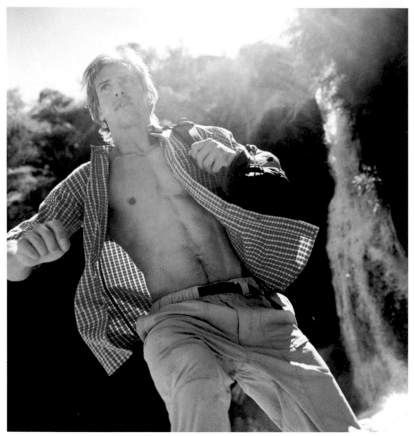

The quintessential abs may look natural, but it takes work to get them – and to keep them.

also responsible for the rippled 'six-pack' or 'shredded' abs look so many guys covet.

Situp

A cousin of the Crunch, the Situp is a very effective exercise for the rectus abdominis, obliques and hip flexors. Situps with your legs straight make your hip flexors work harder than the bent-knee variety, and will bring better overall results.

Crunch

This is a simple floor exercise that works the entire rectus abdominis and the obliques. Contrary to their reputation, however, Crunches alone will not deliver that six-pack – although this much appreciated exercise does assist mightily in abs development and definition. Only aerobic exercise and a fat-burning diet will reveal those much-desired bulges that yearn for development.

Squat

This exercise targets every muscle in your lower body: the quadriceps (a group of four muscles on the front of the thigh responsible for straightening your leg); the hamstrings (very big muscles at the back of the thigh responsible for straightening your torso when it's bent forwards at the hips); the gluteals (the buttocks muscles responsible for jumping and sprinting, which act in tandem with your hamstrings to straighten your hips); and the muscles of the lower back, such as the erector spinae. Plus, it works the muscles in your lower legs, midsection and middle back. If you could pick only one gym exercise for overall body fitness, the Squat would be the one to choose.

Deadlift

Like the Squat, the Deadlift also delivers a lot of benefits in a short amount of time. The Deadlift mar- shals the forces of much of the upper and lower body, using the hamstrings and gluteals as prime movers, but also working your lower-back and trapezius muscles. In fact, everything on the back of your body gets a workout with this one move. The name of the exercise refers to the fact that you are supposed to perform the lift from a stationary position, not relying on any body momentum. The deadlift is difficult and one that requires a level of concentration. It is one of the most dramatic moves in competitive powerlifting.

Lunge

A simple move – bending the knee and moving the body forwards – becomes a reliable lower-body workout when you hold a dumbbell in each hand. The quadriceps, hamstrings and gluteals are targeted by a wide variety of Lunge variations. This exercise is easy to do at home.

GET PUMPED

After a couple of sets, the muscles you're targeting will feel full and hard. This is the pump, and it's the best feeling you can have in a weight room. You can see the results of your work; you look better already. The pump also serves an important physiological purpose. The movements that trap blood in your muscles also generate lactic acid. Lactic acid helps to produce growth hormone, which is believed to help muscles grow bigger and at the same time shrink fat cells by mobilizing fat for energy.

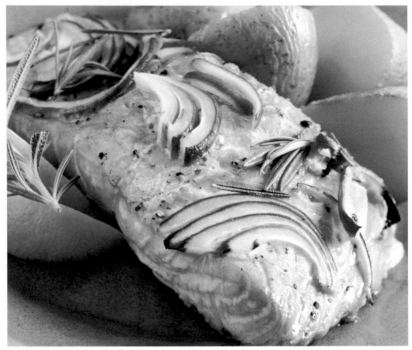

Skip the latest fads and feast on fats – the right ones. They're the fuel that your body needs.

Diet and Nutrition

Dietary fat helps to build muscle, burn body fat, control cholesterol and keep your heart, head and hormones working right. So why are we so afraid to eat it?

In the 1980s, nutritionists everywhere told us if we wanted to stay alive and slim, we could have perhaps a tiny lick of butter once a week, but any more fat and we'd die young and obese. Gone was the simple idea, passed down from generation to generation, that excess carbohydrates will make you fat. Gone, too, was the simplest weight-loss plan ever devised: eat the meat, skip the potatoes.

But the idea that dietary fat by itself causes obesity, once accepted as gospel, has recently been relegated to the status of myth. That's because the world of weight-loss research is beginning what may be the most spectacular about-turn in its history. It seems that some studies lasting a year or more have shown weight gains with low-fat diets. Compensatory mechanisms kick in when the body is presented with a low-fat diet over a long period, and as a result we stop losing weight.

Meanwhile, dietary fat has a satiating effect, meaning you feel fuller longer. Protein, often found in abundance in high-fat foods and generally absent from low-fat foods, does this, and also makes you feel full faster while you're still eating. A mound of rice or a bowl of popcorn has neither effect. You don't feel satisfied, so instead you keep eating.

And after you stop eating, you get hungrier faster.

In other words, there is no benefit to cutting fat from your diet just for the sake of cutting fat. There is no benefit to adding carbohydrates just because they're low in fat. In fact, the combination of these two ideas may end up contributing to more overweight, unhealthy people.

Does that mean you can eat as much bacon or as many cheeseburgers as you want, without worrying about such dire consequences as

LOSE WEIGHT FAST

A crash diet is never a good idea, but there are a few commonsense steps you can take to shed extra kilos quickly.

1. Stop drinking fruit juice. Depending on how much you already drink, it's possible to shed 2.25 kg (5 pounds) in a month simply by dropping juice and sugared sodas from your diet.

2. Go easy with energy bars. And energy gels. And pretty much any of the high-calorie additives that claim to boost your workout. Unless you want to gain weight, the food from your last meal – assuming that you ate it within the past two hours and it was nutritious – should provide all the energy you need for moderate workouts.

3. Make friends with fruits and vegetables. Add a piece of fruit to each meal and an extra portion of vegetables to lunch and dinner. You will feel fuller and eat less at your next snack or meal.

4. Cut out beer. Yes, you heard right. It may be an extreme move, but many guys would actually lose 4.5 kg (10 pounds) in a month if they were able to drop this 'staple' from their diet. If this is too harsh, switch to light beer and settle for dropping 2.25 kg (5 pounds).

weight gain or heart attacks? Well, not exactly.

Not all fat is created equal, and different fats have different effects on your health. Here are the five most common types of fats, listed in descending order of health benefits.

Omega-3 Polyunsaturated Fat

Found in: Fish and fish oil; flaxseeds (linseeds) and flaxseed (linseed) oil

Why you need it: This is an 'essential' fat, meaning your body can't make it from other fats; you have to get some in your diet. It used to be plentiful in the human diet – grass-fed animals had it in their meat, so whenever your great-grandfather

Eating smaller, healthier meals more frequently during the day will help stave off binging.

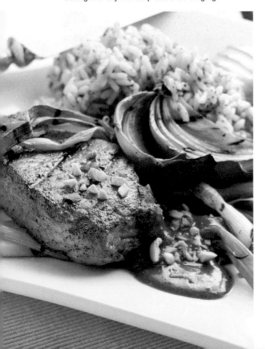

killed and grilled a deer, he got a load of omega-3s. But today's grain-fed livestock have little omega-3 fat. Some researchers think this absence of omega-3s is such a serious problem that symptoms of aging are actually omega-3 deficiencies.

What it does: Lowers triglycerides dramatically, and may also lead to significant fat loss.

Why you want more of it in your diet: A 1997 study showed that 6 grams a day of fish-oil supplements changed the body's metabolism of fat and carbohydrates. Study subjects who took fish oil burned more fat for energy and stored more carbs.

Monounsaturated Fat

Found in: Nuts and seeds; peanut butter; olives and olive oil; avocados

Why you need it: It's not an essential fat, so technically your body can make it from other fats. But it's in most of the fat-rich foods you eat anyway, so you get some whether you mean to or not.

What it does: Lowers total and LDL ('bad') cholesterol; raises HDL ('good') cholesterol; lowers triglycerides; boosts Vitamin E levels.

Why you want more of it in your diet: Monounsaturated fat helps you to burn more fat, especially if you're overweight. It may also lower the risk of coronary heart disease.

Omega-6 Polyunsaturated Fat

Found in: All the vegetable oils used in commercial food processing; meat; eggs; dairy products

Why you need it: Like omega-3s, omega-6 fats are essential, meaning you have to get them from food. But since omega-6 fats are so common in almost everyone's diet, you'd have to eat a virtually fat-free diet to have a deficiency.

What it does: Lowers total and LDL cholesterol; raises HDL cholesterol; lowers triglycerides.

Why you want less of it: Consuming too many omega-6s and too few omega-3s can lead to a long list of unfortunate outcomes. It has been linked to everything from cancer to Alzheimer's Disease.

Saturated Fat

Found in: Meat, dairy products

Why you need it: Technically, you don't. However, saturated fats are important to building cell structures.

What it does: Raises total and LDL cholesterol dramatically; raises HDL cholesterol; lowers triglycerides.

Why you want less of it: Saturated fat seems to be more likely to be stored away in the body than other types of fats. Mono and omega-3 fats seem to be more readily used for energy.

Trans Fat

Found in: Margarine; crisps; bakery products (on food labels, the words 'partially hydrogenated' mean it's a synthesized trans fat).

CRAVING SWEETS?

After a big workout, your glycogen (or stored carbohydrate) levels can drop to zero if you haven't taken in enough calories. That's why you sometimes crave a sweet, high-calorie snack after a session at the gym. A better way to get the energy you need is to work out ahead of time how many calories you should be consuming each day. To calculate your basal metabolic rate (BMR) – the number of calories you need just to survive – use the following formula:

BMR = 66 + (13.7 x weight in kg) + (5 x height in cm) - (6.8 x age in years)

Then, to work out how many calories you need to get through your work day and your workout, use the formula below that best matches your activity level:

Sedentary = BMR x 1.2　　　**Moderately active = BMR x 1.55**
Lightly active = BMR x 1.375　　　**Very active = BMR x 1.725**

What it does: Trans fat (transformed from one type of fat to another) raises total and LDL cholesterol; lowers HDL cholesterol; lowers triglycerides.

Why you want less of it: There's no scientific consensus yet, but some evidence suggests these nasty fats contribute more to cardiovascular disease than any other type of fat.

The key to good nutrition is to eat the best foods in every category. That means foods rich in the good fats, such as lean meat, fish, eggs, olive oil and nuts, along with the best carbohydrates – whole grains, fresh fruits, and fibre- and antioxidant-rich vegetables.

But here's the new twist: build each meal and snack around fat and protein. Then fill out the meal with carbohydrates to add flavour, texture, variety and colour.

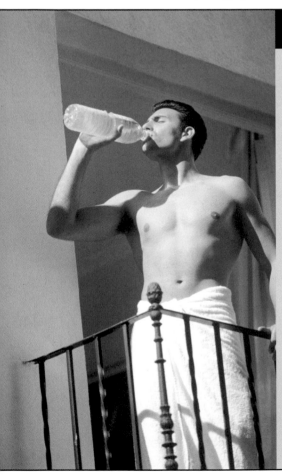

STAY HYDRATED

A fit, 82 kg (180-pound) man who lifts weights for one hour will burn approximately 490 calories (2,051 kJ) – and lose about 240 ml (8 ounces) of water. Dehydration can lead to a drop in blood pressure, a heightened pulse rate and increased fatigue, which can really interfere with your progress. In general, it's advisable to drink 480 ml (16 ounces) of water two hours before working out.

If you're on a high-protein diet, you'll need to drink even more, because people on higher protein diets store less water in their bodies. You can avoid problems by drinking more fluids – at least two to three glasses more than the recommended eight glasses a day.

EAT MORE, LOSE MORE

Here's the typical weight-loss formula: eat less. It works for a while – 2.4 days, to be exact – and then you're back on all fours, shoving hamburgers down your throat like a supermodel on her birthday. The key to weight loss isn't depriving yourself all the time; it's eating the foods that will keep you full. Start here:

Add fat. Just make sure it's the monounsaturated type, such as olive oil or peanut butter.

Add snacks. But they should be foods with a low glycaemic index, meaning they won't cause your insulin levels to spike and your hunger to follow. Try low-fat chocolate milk, peanuts or low-fat yogurt.

Add carbohydrates. But moderately. If you eat a snack or have a lunch that's rich in carbohydrates, your body will release serotonin, a feel-good chemical. But in a couple of hours, those levels will drop – and you'll be more likely to binge. Try light popcorn to keep your serotonin levels even.

A Muscle-Building Meal Plan

Muscle happens all day, every day. After one good workout, your body will spend the next 48 to 72 hours building and repairing your muscle cells. The least you can do is give it the best materials to work with – high-quality protein to build and repair muscles, the most nutrient-dense carbohydrates to provide energy and heart-healthy unsaturated fats to help you feel full longer.

But instead of giving your body three big meals a day, you're going to eat six smaller meals. Frequent small meals can help prevent your love handles from developing, and keep your body from tapping into your muscle protein for energy during workouts or between meals.

On the next two pages, you'll find a plan for one day of healthy eating. Use the logic in the plan to create meals that will keep you fit and fuelled. And be sure to add a glass of water (240 ml, 8 oz) at 9:30 am, 12:45 pm, and 3:15 pm – in addition to the water you drink with your meals.

This meal plan has 3,080 calories (12,892 kJ) for a thin guy who wants to add size to his frame. If you want to lose weight, cut down to about 2,000 calories (8,372 kJ) a day (still distributed over six meals). If you want to lose fat and gain muscle, aim for 2,700 calories (11,302 kJ) a day.

MEAL 1
8 A.M.

3 eggs
75 g (2½ oz) oatmeal with
145 g (5 oz) blueberries
240 ml (8 fl oz) skimmed
milk

Add a multivitamin/mineral
supplement that supplies
100 per cent of the daily
requirements for the
majority of vitamins and
minerals listed on its label.

**What you can eat
instead:** Swap the oatmeal
and berries for a high-fibre
cereal with raisins and
an orange. Cottage cheese
or three low-fat turkey
sausages can fill in for the
eggs.

MEAL 2
11 A.M.

A tuna sandwich with
salad. . .

½ tin (75 g) tuna (use
    white or light tuna
    packed in water; drain
    the water), mixed with
    1 t (5 ml) mayonnaise
2 slices wholegrain bread
2 handfuls mixed salad
    (dark green lettuce,
    carrots, chopped peppers
    (capsicums), tomatoes
    and onions are all good)
1 T (15 ml) olive oil in
    whatever dressing you
    choose (that much olive
    oil contains 14 g of fat).
    If you're using a bottled
    dressing containing olive
    oil, use whatever serving
    size gets you to 14 g
1 large orange (eaten
    separately or as part of
    the salad)

**What you can eat
instead:** Swap the tuna for
a lean roast beef sandwich
with wholegrain mustard. If
you get sick of the greens,
quarter two tomatoes and
mix them with a handful of
chickpeas, some chopped
fresh basil and a teaspoon
(5 ml) of olive oil. Half a
cantaloupe will stand in
nicely for the orange.

MEAL 3
2 P.M.

A chicken sandwich. . .

90 g (3 oz) sliced chicken
breast
2 slices wholegrain bread
1 T (15 ml) mayonnaise

Add some lettuce, and
sliced green pepper (cap-
sicum), onion or tomato.

**What you can eat
instead:** Any kind of lean
meat will be fine in a
sandwich. Or try a big
(480 ml, 16-oz) tin of soup
– minestrone, for example
– and add 90 g (3 oz) of
cooked turkey or chicken.

RECIPE KEY

T = Tablespoon
t = teaspoon
g = gram
ml = millilitre

MEAL 4
(PREWORKOUT)
4:30 P.M.

A shake or smoothie. . .

1 scoop (about 20 g) whey protein powder
240 ml (8 fl oz) skimmed milk
145 g (5 oz) fresh or frozen berries
240 ml (8 fl oz) orange juice
1 t (5 ml) flaxseed (linseed) oil (keep refrigerated)
1 t (5 ml) olive oil

What you can eat instead: Try 240 ml (8 fl oz) of skimmed milk, an apple and either 30 g (1 oz) of nuts or 2 T (30 g) of peanut butter. You'll be light on protein, so you'll need to add 30 g (1 oz) of chicken or turkey breast to the previous meal and 30 g (1 oz) of salmon to the next.

MEAL 5
(POST WORKOUT)
6:45 P.M.

Another shake or smoothie. . .

1½ scoops (about 30 g) whey protein powder
480 ml (16 fl oz) fruit juice

What you can eat instead: Try 480 ml (16 fl oz) of plain nonfat yogurt blended with 145 g (5 oz) of strawberries.

MEAL 6
8:30 P.M.

170 g (6 oz) salmon, grilled or poached
1 medium baked sweet potato
145 g (5 oz) brown rice
2 handfuls salad (with the same ingredients as previously)
1 T (15 ml) olive oil in the dressing of your choice

What you can eat instead: Any type of lean meat – steak, pork loin, chicken breast. Instead of sweet potatoes, try a banana, dried apricots or dried figs.

Chicken is a quick, healthy and satisfying alternative to heavier fare.

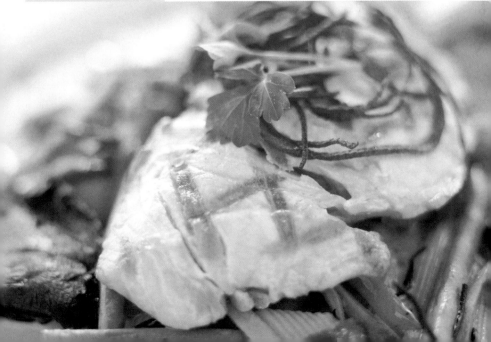

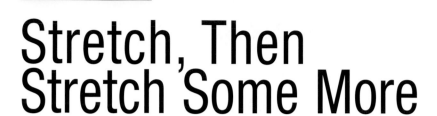

Stretch, Then Stretch Some More

You probably don't want to be reminded of this, but by the time most guys reach adulthood, many of their muscles have significantly tightened. Before any workout, it is important to stretch every major muscle group in your body. You need to be completely warmed up before you lift. Working out with cold, tight muscles increases your risk of injury. Here are some essential stretches that will make sure you bend instead of break. Two things to remember: first, never stretch cold muscles; always do 5 to 10 minutes of light aerobic exercise beforehand. Secondly, don't hold your breath while you stretch.

TOWEL TRICEPS STRETCH
Targets: Deltoids, Triceps

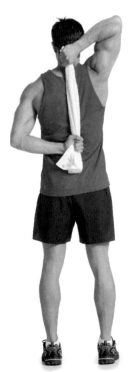

Holding one end of a towel in each hand, place your right hand behind your head and your left hand at the small of your back. Gently pull down with your left hand until you feel a tug or tension in your right shoulder and triceps. Hold this stretch for 15 to 30 seconds, then gently pull up with your right hand until you feel a tug or tension in your left shoulder. Hold for 15 to 30 seconds. Switch hands and repeat.

UPPER-BACK STRETCH
Targets: Rhomboids, Trapezius

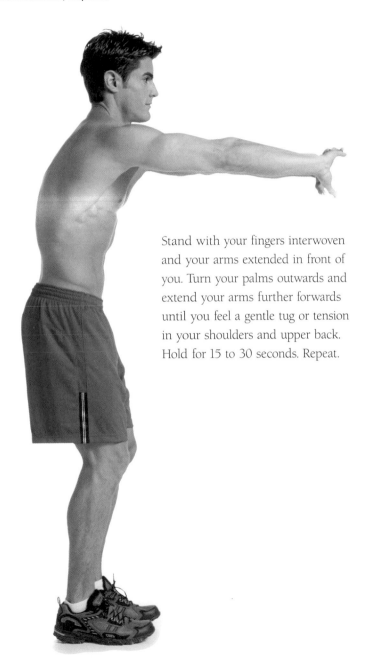

Stand with your fingers interwoven and your arms extended in front of you. Turn your palms outwards and extend your arms further forwards until you feel a gentle tug or tension in your shoulders and upper back. Hold for 15 to 30 seconds. Repeat.

CHEST STRETCH
Targets: Pectoralis Major, Anterior Deltoids

Stand with your fingers interwoven behind your back.
Extend your arms up behind
you until you feel a gentle tug
or tension in your shoulders
and chest. Hold this stretch for
15 to 30 seconds. Repeat.

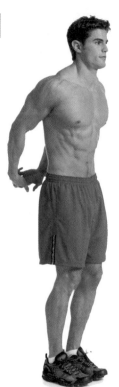

ABDOMINAL STRETCH
Targets: Abdominals, Hip Flexors, Chest, Front Shoulders

Lie flat on your stomach. Slowly (repeat: slowly) lift your chest off the floor.
The idea is not to strain your neck, but to gently lift your upper body. At the
same time, raise your lower legs off the floor about 3 centimetres. Extend
your hands behind you, as if you were trying to stretch your fingertips to
your heels. Hold this stretch for 15 to 30 seconds.

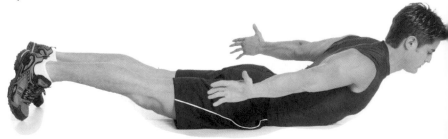

HIP FLEXOR STRETCH

Targets: Hip Flexors, Abdominals (first position); Hip Flexors, Obliques (second position)

Kneel on your left knee on a pad or carpeted floor, with your left knee almost a metre behind your right heel. Start with your torso upright, arms straight out and parallel to the floor, palms forwards. Lean back until you feel a good stretch in your left hip flexors. Hold 10 to 20 seconds (balance could be an issue), repeat, then switch legs and do the same. You can also try the stretch to the side, instead of leaning back, to work your obliques.

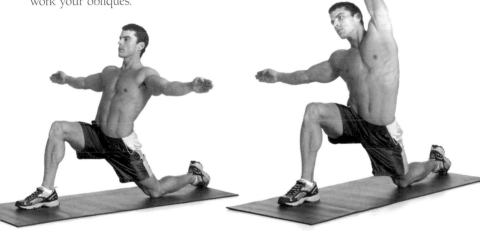

GROIN STRETCH

Targets: Adductor Longus

Sit on the floor. Place the soles of your feet together, with your hands on your ankles. Gently move your hips forwards until you feel a gentle tension in the groin. Hold this stretch for 15 to 30 seconds. Repeat.

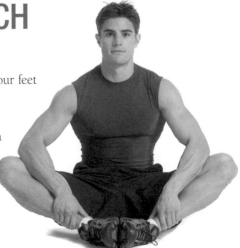

FULL-BODY STRETCH

Targets: Calves, Hamstrings, Hips, Knees, Glutes, Lower-Back Muscles, Shoulder and Wrist

Sit on the floor with your left leg extended. Bring the sole of your right foot against the inside of your left thigh. Slowly and gently, bend forwards from the hips, reaching your fingers towards your left foot until you feel a slight tug or tension. Hold this stretch for 15 to 30 seconds. Bend forwards twice more, holding the stretch for 15 to 30 seconds. Stop if you feel pain. Repeat with your right leg extended.

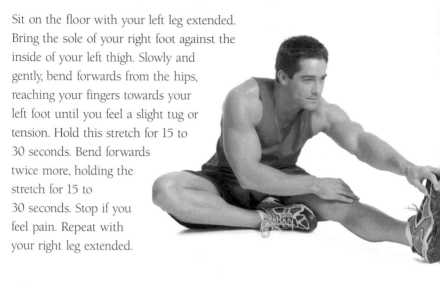

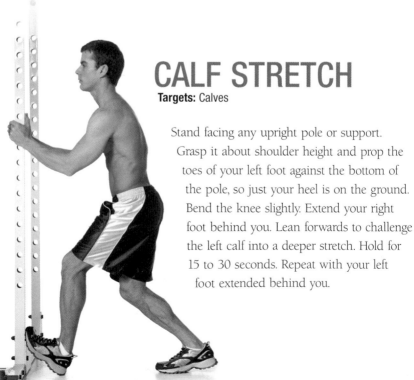

CALF STRETCH

Targets: Calves

Stand facing any upright pole or support. Grasp it about shoulder height and prop the toes of your left foot against the bottom of the pole, so just your heel is on the ground. Bend the knee slightly. Extend your right foot behind you. Lean forwards to challenge the left calf into a deeper stretch. Hold for 15 to 30 seconds. Repeat with your left foot extended behind you.

PART II:
The Exercises

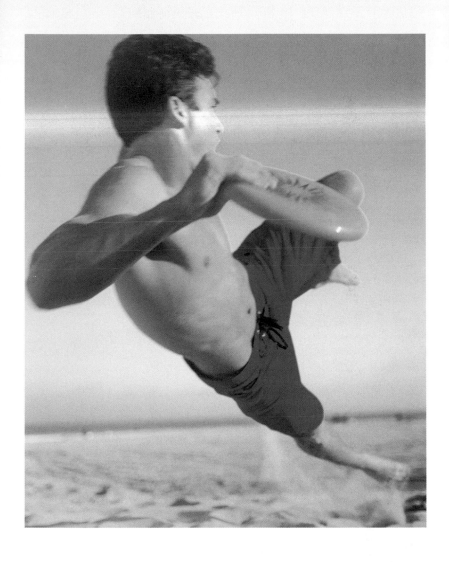

Chest, Back and Arms

Essential upper-body exercises for total-body fitness

Ready? Here are the 15 best exercises in even more detail, with plenty of variations. They focus on all the major muscle groups, generally from top to bottom. These descriptions will teach you the proper form and rhythm for each move. Look for tips along the way that will polish your form and help to prevent injury.

MAIN
PRESS-UP

Targets: Pectorals, Abdominals, Triceps

▉ Kneel on the floor with your hands about shoulder-width apart. Stretch your legs straight behind you, letting your body weight rest on your palms and toes. Keep your back straight by tucking your pelvis and keep your head even with your shoulders. Don't let your head drop or strain backwards.

TRAINER'S TIP

Make the press-ups harder by having a spotter place a weighted plate on your back between your shoulder blades. Start with about 4.5 kilograms.

▉ Slowly lower yourself until your chest touches the floor.

▉ Pause at the bottom, then return to the starting position.

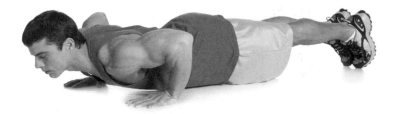

PRESS-UP VARIANT
PLYOMETRIC PRESS-UP
Targets: Pectorals, Abdominals, Triceps

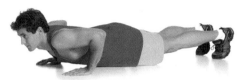

1 Assume the basic Press-up position on a well-padded carpet or exercise mat.

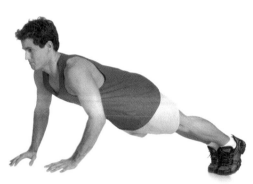

2 Lower yourself to the bottom position, then quickly push up with enough force so your hands come off the floor.

3 Catch yourself with your elbows slightly bent, lower to the bottom position, and push immediately into the next repetition.

PRESS-UP VARIANT
THREE-POINT PRESS-UP
Targets: Pectorals, Abdominals, Triceps

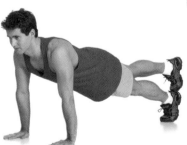

1 Assume the basic Press-up position, with one difference: place one foot on the heel of the other, so that your body is positioned on three points.

TRAINER'S TIP

This press-up works your muscles more intensely, because it distributes your weight on three points instead of four.

2 Slowly lower your body to the floor, pause, and push yourself back up. Switch legs halfway through your set.

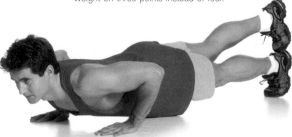

MAIN
CURL
Target: Biceps

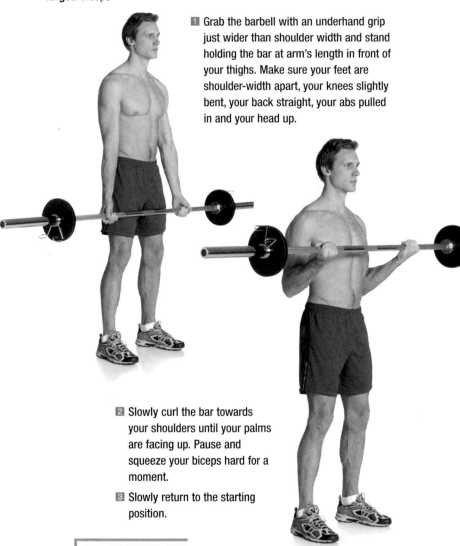

1. Grab the barbell with an underhand grip just wider than shoulder width and stand holding the bar at arm's length in front of your thighs. Make sure your feet are shoulder-width apart, your knees slightly bent, your back straight, your abs pulled in and your head up.

2. Slowly curl the bar towards your shoulders until your palms are facing up. Pause and squeeze your biceps hard for a moment.

3. Slowly return to the starting position.

TRAINER'S TIP

Proper stance will prevent you from leaning back to help lift the weight. Keeping your upper arms close to your sides will prevent you from swinging your arms to help the lift.

CURL VARIANT
STANDING DUMBBELL BICEPS CURL
Target: Biceps

1 Stand holding the dumbbells at arm's length slightly in front of you with an underhand grip.

2 Keeping your upper arms against your sides, curl the weights towards your shoulders (both at the same time) until your palms are facing up.

3 Hold your arms in the topmost position for a moment, then slowly return to the starting position.

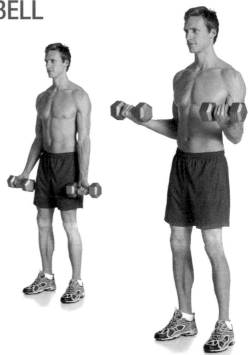

CURL VARIANT
CABLE BICEPS CURL
Target: Biceps

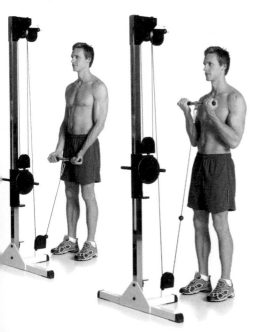

1 Attach a straight bar to the low pulley of a cable station. Grab the bar with a shoulder-width, underhand grip and hold it at arm's length just in front of your thighs. Stand straight with your upper arms tucked against your sides. Your feet should be hip-width apart, knees slightly bent.

2 Curl the bar towards your chest as far as you can without letting your upper arms move.

3 Pause, then slowly return to the starting position.

CURL VARIANT
TRICEPS PUSH-DOWN
Targets: Triceps

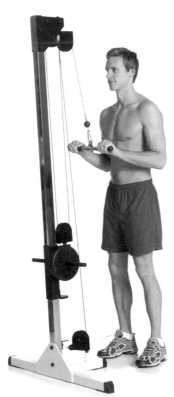

1 Attach a straight bar to a high pulley. Grab the bar with an overhand grip, keeping your hands 15 to 30 centimetres apart. Stand with about 30 centimetres between you and the weight stack, tuck your elbows close to your sides and pull the bar down until your forearms are just above parallel to the floor.

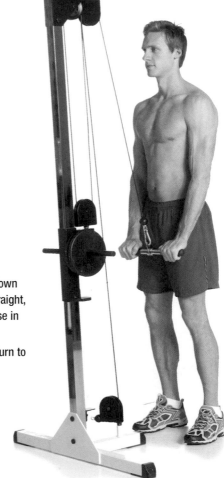

2 Slowly push the bar down until your arms are straight, keeping everything else in the original position.

3 Pause, then slowly return to the starting position.

CURL VARIANT
LYING PULL-OVER
Targets: Long Head of Triceps, Latissimus Dorsi, Lower Chest

1 Grab an EZ-curl bar with an overhand grip just inside shoulder width. Lie on your back on a flat bench. With your elbows bent about 90 degrees, hold the bar over your chest.

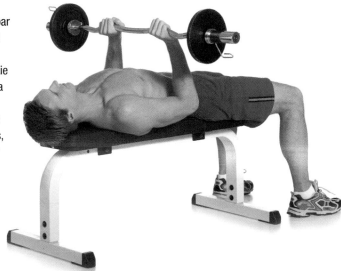

2 Lower the bar back behind your head, until your upper arms are roughly parallel to the floor. Then pull the bar back to the starting position.

3 For more emphasis on the triceps, try this exercise with straight or nearly straight arms.

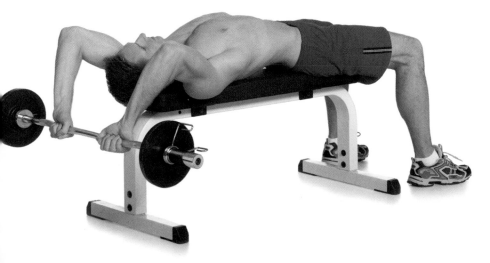

CURL VARIANT
LYING TRICEPS EXTENSION
Targets: Triceps

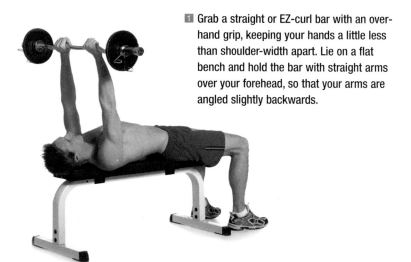

1 Grab a straight or EZ-curl bar with an over-hand grip, keeping your hands a little less than shoulder-width apart. Lie on a flat bench and hold the bar with straight arms over your forehead, so that your arms are angled slightly backwards.

2 Without moving your upper arms, bend your elbows to lower the bar as far as you can. (Do this slowly and carefully; there's a reason the exercise is sometimes called a 'skull crusher'.)

3 Pause, then straighten your arms to lift the weights back to the starting position.

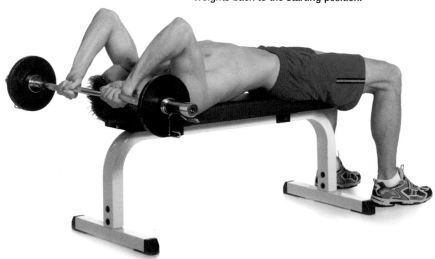

MAIN
BARBELL BENCH PRESS

Targets: Pectorals, Triceps

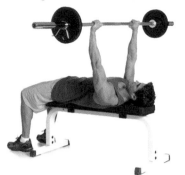

1. Lie on a bench with your feet wide and flat on the floor. Grab the barbell with an overhand grip. Place your hands just beyond shoulder-width apart. Start with the barbell straight up over your chest while pulling your shoulder blades back towards each other.

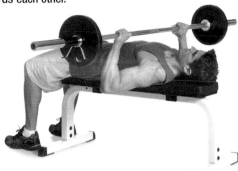

2. Lower the bar – slowly – to the middle of your chest. Then push it straight up over your chest again. Keep your shoulder blades pulled together throughout the movement.

MAIN
SHOULDER PRESS

Targets: Deltoids, Triceps, Lower Trapezius

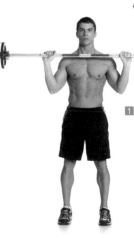

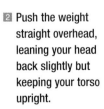

1. Grab a barbell with a shoulder-width, overhand grip. Stand holding the barbell at shoulder level, your feet shoulder-width apart and knees slightly bent.

2. Push the weight straight overhead, leaning your head back slightly but keeping your torso upright.

3. Pause, then slowly lower the bar to the starting position.

SHOULDER PRESS VARIANT
SEATED BARBELL SHOULDER PRESS

Targets: Deltoids, Triceps, Trapezius

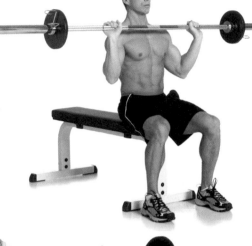

1 Grab a barbell with an over-hand grip that's shoulder-width or a little wider. Sit on the end of a bench with your feet flat on the floor.

2 Hold the bar at collar-bone level and keep your back in a neutral position. Press the barbell overhead until your arms are straight but your elbows are not locked.

3 Slowly return the bar to collarbone level.

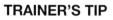

TRAINER'S TIP

Don't lean back; keep your torso straight, and only move your head enough to avoid hitting yourself with the bar-bell. If you have to lean, the weight is too heavy.

SHOULDER PRESS VARIANT
FRENCH PRESS
Targets: Triceps

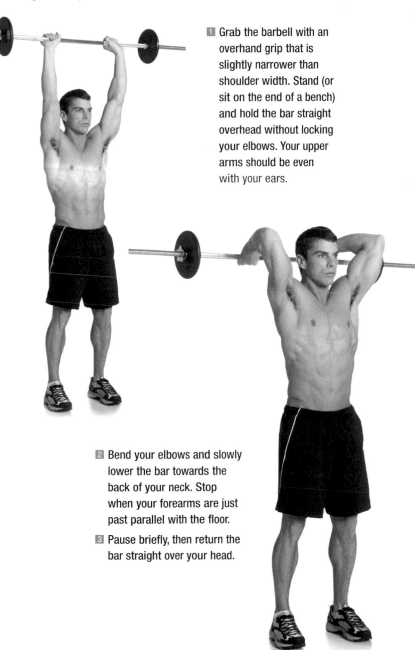

1 Grab the barbell with an overhand grip that is slightly narrower than shoulder width. Stand (or sit on the end of a bench) and hold the bar straight overhead without locking your elbows. Your upper arms should be even with your ears.

2 Bend your elbows and slowly lower the bar towards the back of your neck. Stop when your forearms are just past parallel with the floor.

3 Pause briefly, then return the bar straight over your head.

MAIN
DIP

Targets: Triceps, Pectorals, Front-Shoulder Deltoids

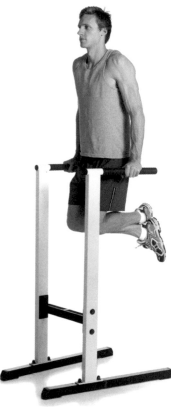

1 Grab the parallel bars of a dip station with a neutral grip and lift yourself so your arms are straight but not locked. Bend your knees and cross your ankles.

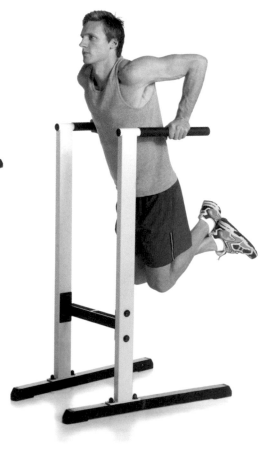

2 Slowly lower your body by bending your elbows until your upper arms are parallel to the floor. (The further you lower yourself, the harder your deltoids work to push you back up.)

3 Pause, then push yourself back to the starting position.

DIP VARIANT
BENCH DIP
Targets: Triceps, Pectorals, Front-Shoulder Deltoids

1 Sit on the edge of a bench or chair and place your palms (fingers to the front) on the bench next to your hips. Extend your legs straight out in front of you. Straighten your arms and move your torso forwards so your buttocks and back are just in front (and clear) of the bench.

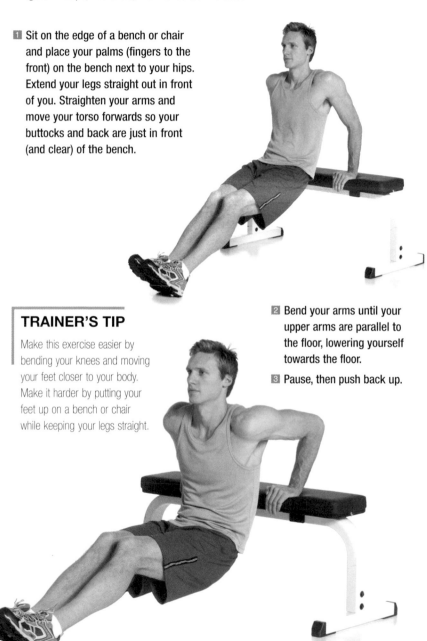

TRAINER'S TIP

Make this exercise easier by bending your knees and moving your feet closer to your body. Make it harder by putting your feet up on a bench or chair while keeping your legs straight.

2 Bend your arms until your upper arms are parallel to the floor, lowering yourself towards the floor.

3 Pause, then push back up.

DIP VARIANT
WEIGHTED DIP
Targets: Triceps, Pectoralis Major, Front-Shoulder Deltoids

1 Attach a weighted belt to your waist and grab the bars of a dip station. Lift yourself so your arms are fully extended. Bend your knees and cross your ankles behind you.

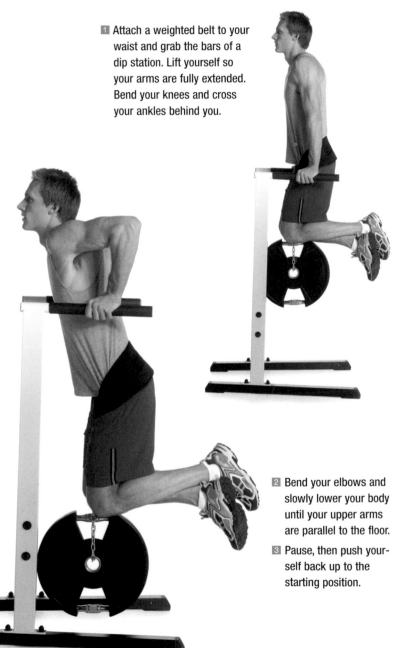

2 Bend your elbows and slowly lower your body until your upper arms are parallel to the floor.

3 Pause, then push yourself back up to the starting position.

MAIN
CABLE ROW
Targets: Upper and Mid-Back, Biceps

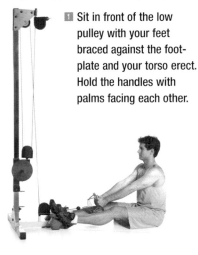

1 Sit in front of the low pulley with your feet braced against the footplate and your torso erect. Hold the handles with palms facing each other.

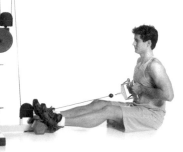

2 Pull your shoulder blades together while steadily pulling the handles towards your abdomen.

3 Pause, then slowly return to the starting position.

CABLE ROW VARIANT
BARBELL BENT-OVER ROW
Targets: Upper and Mid-Back, Biceps

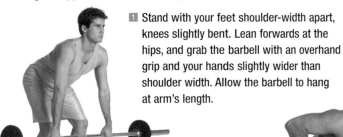

1 Stand with your feet shoulder-width apart, knees slightly bent. Lean forwards at the hips, and grab the barbell with an overhand grip and your hands slightly wider than shoulder width. Allow the barbell to hang at arm's length.

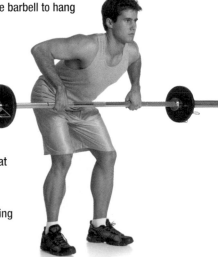

2 Pull the bar up to your abdomen without raising your torso, keeping your hips bent at the same angle throughout the lift.

3 Pause with the bar at your abdomen, then slowly return to the starting position, keeping your torso at the same angle.

CABLE ROW VARIANT
DUMBBELL BENT-OVER ROW
Targets: Upper and Mid-Back, Biceps

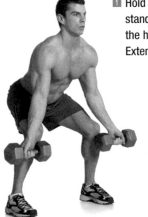

1 Hold a pair of dumbbells with an underhand grip, standing with your knees bent. Bend forwards at the hips with your lower back slightly arched. Extend your arms towards the floor.

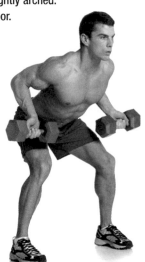

2 Pull the dumbbells up to the sides of your torso, until your elbows are slightly higher than your torso.

3 Pause, then lower the dumbbells back towards the floor.

CABLE ROW VARIANT
CABLE UPRIGHT ROW
Targets: Trapezius, Deltoids, Biceps

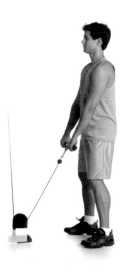
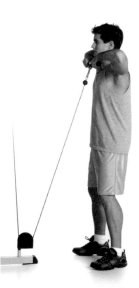

1 Attach a straight bar to the low cable. Stand with about 30 centimetres between you and the weight stack and grab the bar with an over-hand, shoulder-width grip. Hold the bar at arm's length in front of your thighs.

2 Pull the bar up until your upper arms are parallel to the floor, or slightly higher.

3 Pause, then lower the bar back to the starting position.

CABLE ROW VARIANT
PISTON UPRIGHT ROW
Targets: Trapezius, Deltoids, Biceps

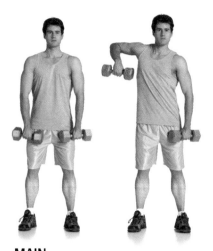

1 Grab a pair of dumbbells with an overhand grip and hold them shoulder-width apart, at arm's length next to your thighs. Stand with your feet shoulder-width apart and your knees slightly bent.

2 Pull your right arm up until the upper arm is parallel to the floor and the dumbbell is up next to your ribs. Without pausing, lower the weight while raising your left arm. Continue pumping out repetitions until you finish the set.

MAIN
FLY
Targets: Pectorals

1 Lie on a bench, holding a pair of dumbbells with a neutral grip (palms facing each other) or overhand grip (palms facing towards your feet) above the middle of your pecs, arms straight up. Maintaining a slight bend in your elbows, lower the dumbbells in an arc down and back until your upper arms are parallel to the floor and in line with your ears.

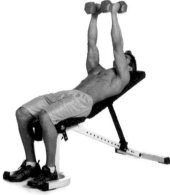

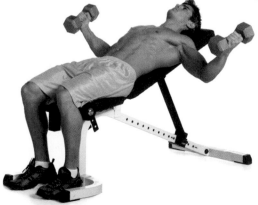

2 Use your chest to pull the weights back up to the starting position, following the same arc-like route in reverse.

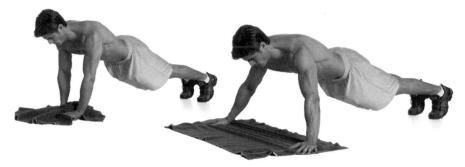

FLY VARIANT
TOWEL CHEST FLY
Targets: Pectorals

1. Place your hands on towels or socks on a smooth floor, your body in position for a press-up. Start with your hands close together.

2. Slide your hands out to your sides to lower your body.

3. Slide your hands back towards each other to return to the starting position.

MAIN
OVERHAND PULL-UP
Targets: Upper and Mid-Back, Biceps

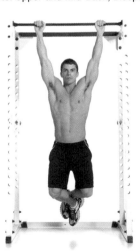

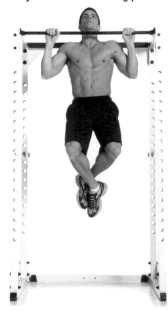

2. Pull yourself up as high as you can.

3. Hold yourself there for a moment, then slowly return to the starting position.

1. Grab the pull-up bar with an overhand grip, your hands slightly wider than your shoulders and hang with your knees bent and ankles crossed.

OVERHAND PULL-UP VARIANT
WEIGHTED PULL-UP
Targets: Upper and Mid-Back, Biceps

Do a regular
Overhand Pull-up
while wearing a
weighted belt,
bumbag or
backpack.

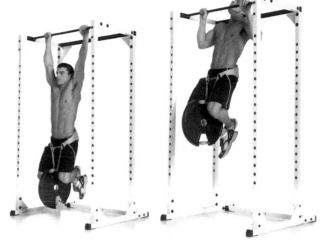

OVERHAND PULL-UP VARIANT
STERNUM PULL-UP
Targets: Upper and Mid-Back, Biceps

Use an underhand grip to grab the bar. Pull
your chest up to the bar and lean back to
give your middle-back an extra workout.

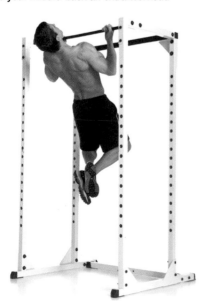

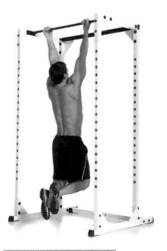

TRAINER'S TIP

On all the Pull-up and Crunch exercises,
exhale as you go up and inhale as you
come down. Always use slow, controlled
movements and don't bounce or jerk.

OVERHAND PULL-UP VARIANT
NEUTRAL-GRIP PULL-UP
Targets: Upper and Mid-Back, Biceps

Take the triangle handle from a cable station and set it over the chin-up bar. Pull yourself up to the right side, then the left, alternating until you finish the set. Start your next set by pulling yourself up to the left.

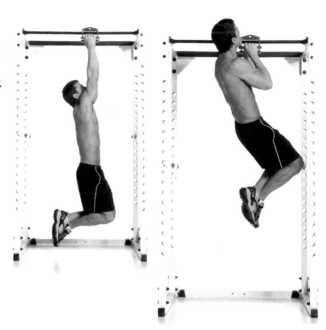

OVERHAND PULL-UP VARIANT
STATIC HANG
Targets: Upper and Mid-Back, Biceps

Grab a pull-up bar with an overhand grip as if you were about to do a Pull-up. Then just... hang. Hold the position for as long as you can (but stop short of muscle failure).

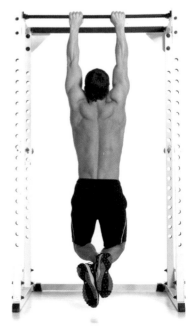

MAIN
BACK EXTENSION
Targets: Hamstrings, Gluteals, Lower Back

1 Position yourself on the back extension station with both feet hooked under the anchor and your arms clasped behind your head. Lower your upper body (allowing your back to round) until it is almost perpendicular to the floor.

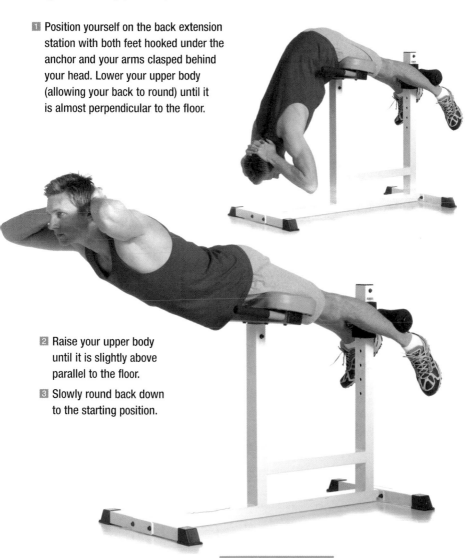

2 Raise your upper body until it is slightly above parallel to the floor.

3 Slowly round back down to the starting position.

TRAINER'S TIP

It's important to engage your core muscles when doing the exercise. This will help to protect your back from injury.

BACK EXTENSION VARIANT
SINGLE-LEG BACK EXTENSION
Targets: Hamstrings, Gluteals, Lower Back

1 Position yourself in the back extension station with one foot hooked under the anchor and the other raised with the knee bent. Clasp your arms behind your head. Lower your upper body until it is almost perpendicular to the floor.

2 Raise your upper body until it is slightly above parallel to the floor.

3 Slowly return to the starting position. Switch feet after completing the set.

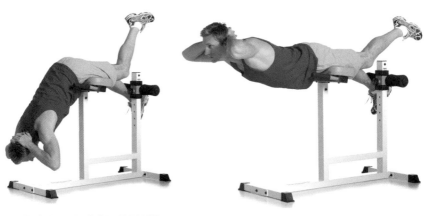

BACK EXTENSION VARIANT
SUPERMAN
Targets: Lower Back

1 Lie face down with your toes on the floor, and your arms stretched out above your head.

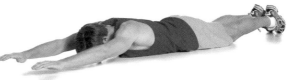

2 Lift your arms, head, chest and lower legs off the floor at the same time, as high as is comfortable for you. Stay in this position for 1 to 5 seconds.

3 Lower everything back to the starting position.

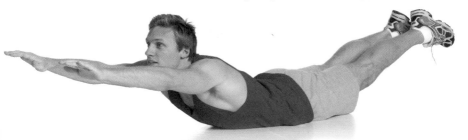

Abdominals

The six-pack crunch, lift and twist

MAIN
HANGING KNEE RAISE

Targets: Abdominals, Hip Flexors, Obliques

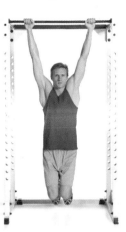 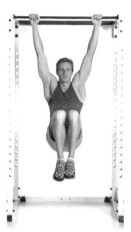

1 Grab a pull-up bar with an overhand grip and hang with your knees bent.

2 Using your lower abdominal muscles, pull your hips up and curl them in towards your chest. Try to lift your knees as close to your chest as you can.

3 Pause and feel the contraction in your lower abs. Slowly return to the starting position.

HANGING KNEE RAISE VARIANT
HANGING KNEE RAISE WITH DIP STATION

Targets: Abdominals, Hip Flexors, Obliques, Biceps, Triceps

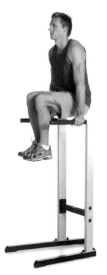 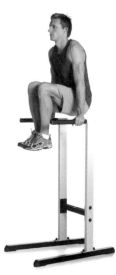

1 Grab the parallel bars of a dip station with a neutral grip and lift yourself so your arms are straight but not locked. Using the muscles of your lower abdominals, pull your hips up and curl them in towards your chest. Try to lift your knees as close to your chest as you can.

2 Pause and feel the contraction in your lower abs. Slowly return your legs to the starting position.

HANGING KNEE RAISE VARIANT
OBLIQUE HANGING KNEE RAISE
Targets: Abdominals, Hip Flexors, Obliques

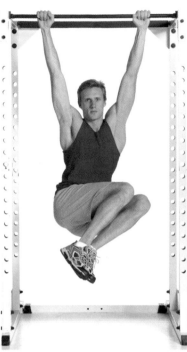

1️⃣ Grab a pull-up bar with an overhand grip and hang from it at arm's length. Raise your legs until your knees are bent at a 90-degree angle.

2️⃣ Keep your knees bent and lift your left hip towards your left armpit, until your lower legs are nearly parallel to the floor.

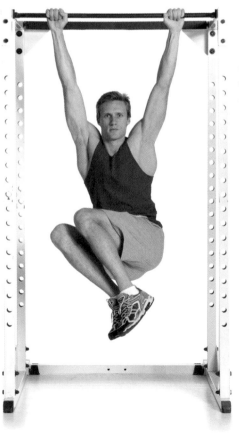

3️⃣ Pause, then return to the bent-knee position. Lift your right hip towards your right armpit. Return to the bent-knee position.

TRAINER'S TIP

The Oblique Hanging Knee Raise may cause discomfort if you have back problems. If you can't do this exercise, try the Swiss Ball Jackknife (page 58) instead.

MAIN
CRUNCH
Targets: Abdominals, Obliques

1 Lie on your back with your feet flat on the floor and your knees bent. Fold your arms loosely across your chest or hold your hands with your fingertips lightly touching behind your ears.

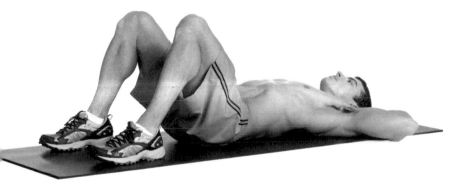

2 Use your abdominal muscles to lift your head and upper torso off the floor while keeping your lower back firmly pressed down.

3 Pause when your shoulder blades are about 5 centimetres off the floor, then slowly return to the starting position.

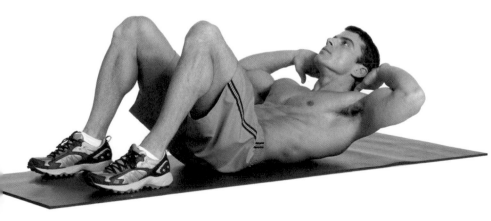

CRUNCH VARIANT
REVERSE CRUNCH
Targets: Abdominals, Hip Flexors

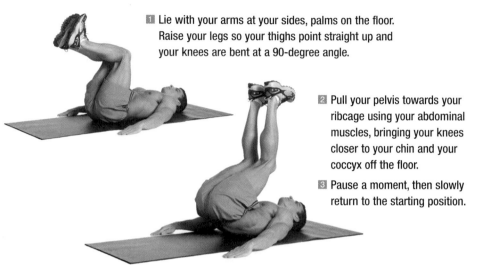

1 Lie with your arms at your sides, palms on the floor. Raise your legs so your thighs point straight up and your knees are bent at a 90-degree angle.

2 Pull your pelvis towards your ribcage using your abdominal muscles, bringing your knees closer to your chin and your coccyx off the floor.

3 Pause a moment, then slowly return to the starting position.

CRUNCH VARIANT
TWISTING CRUNCH
Targets: Obliques

1 Lie on your back with your knees bent and your feet flat on the floor. Put your fingers lightly behind your head.

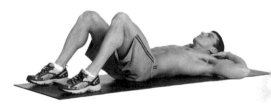

2 Slowly curl your right shoulder towards your left knee until your right shoulder blade just comes off the floor. Hold for a few seconds and concentrate on squeezing your abs tightly.

3 Return slowly to the starting position, then repeat by bringing your left shoulder to your right knee.

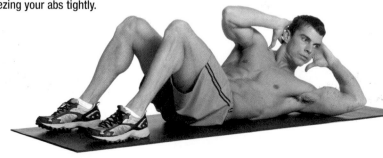

CRUNCH VARIANT
SIDE CRUNCH
Targets: Obliques

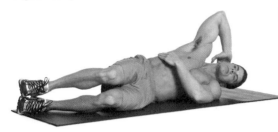

1 Lie on your left side with your left arm across your chest and your right hand lightly touching your head behind your ear.

2 Crunch your right armpit towards your right hip.

3 Pause, then return to the starting position. Repeat on the other side.

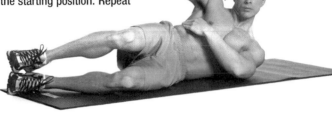

CRUNCH VARIANT
INCLINE REVERSE CRUNCH
Targets: Abdominals, Hip Flexors

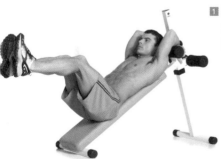

1 Lie on a slant board with your hips lower than your head and your knees slightly bent. Grasp the bar behind you.

2 Pull your hips upwards and inwards, as if you were emptying a bucket of water that rested on your pelvis. Keep your knees at the same angle throughout the movement.

3 Pause, then slowly lower your hips to the starting position.

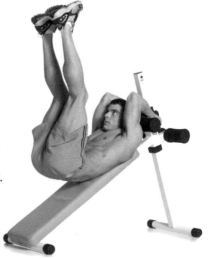

CRUNCH VARIANT
WEIGHTED CRUNCH

Targets: Abdominals, Obliques

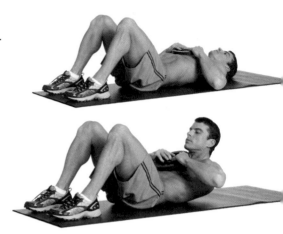

1 Lie on the floor in the Crunch position, holding a dumbbell or weight plate on your upper chest just below your chin.

2 Use your abdominal muscles to lift your head and upper torso off the floor while keeping your lower back firmly pressed down.

3 Pause when your shoulder blades are slightly off the floor, then slowly return to the starting position.

CRUNCH VARIANT
SWISS BALL JACKKNIFE

Targets: Abdominals, Hip Flexors, Obliques

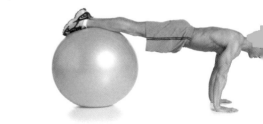

1 Get into Press-up position – your hands set slightly wider than your shoulders – but instead of placing your feet on the floor, rest your shins on a Swiss ball.

2 Keep your arms straight and your back flat.

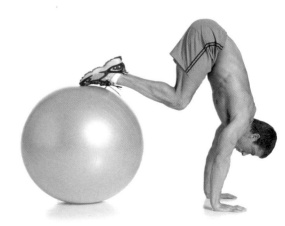

3 Roll the Swiss ball towards your chest by raising your hips and rounding your back as you pull the ball forwards with your feet.

4 Pause, then return the ball to the starting position by rolling it backwards.

MAIN
SITUP

Targets: Abdominals, Obliques, Hip Flexors

1. Holding a dumbbell or other light weight on your chest with both hands, lie on your back on the floor, your knees bent and feet flat on the floor.

2. Slowly lift your torso by curling your upper body towards your knees.

3. Pause, then slowly lower your torso without resting your back on the floor.

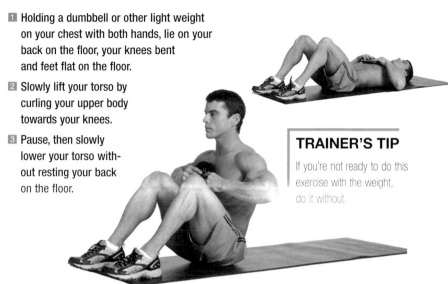

TRAINER'S TIP

If you're not ready to do this exercise with the weight, do it without.

SITUP VARIANT
V-UP

Targets: Abdominals, Hip Flexors, Obliques

1. Lie on your back on the floor with your legs straight. Hold your arms straight above your chest, with your fingers pointing straight out.

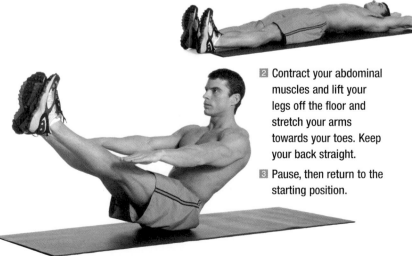

2. Contract your abdominal muscles and lift your legs off the floor and stretch your arms towards your toes. Keep your back straight.

3. Pause, then return to the starting position.

Legs

Build a strong, supple lower body

MAIN

DUMBBELL SQUAT

Targets: Gluteals, Quadriceps, Hamstrings, Lower Back

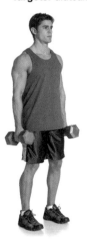

1 Stand holding a pair of dumb-bells down at your sides with a neutral grip, your feet shoulder-width apart. Pull your shoulder blades towards each other.

2 Bend your knees and lower your body as though you were sitting down on a short stool, stopping when your thighs are parallel to the floor.

3 Slowly stand back up to the starting position.

SQUAT VARIANT

FRONT SQUAT

Targets: Gluteals, Quadriceps, Hamstrings, Lower Back

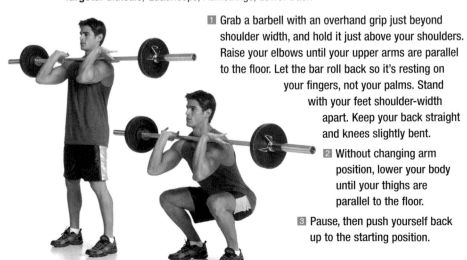

1 Grab a barbell with an overhand grip just beyond shoulder width, and hold it just above your shoulders. Raise your elbows until your upper arms are parallel to the floor. Let the bar roll back so it's resting on your fingers, not your palms. Stand with your feet shoulder-width apart. Keep your back straight and knees slightly bent.

2 Without changing arm position, lower your body until your thighs are parallel to the floor.

3 Pause, then push yourself back up to the starting position.

SQUAT VARIANT
ZERCHER SQUAT
Targets: Lower Back, Hamstrings, Quadriceps

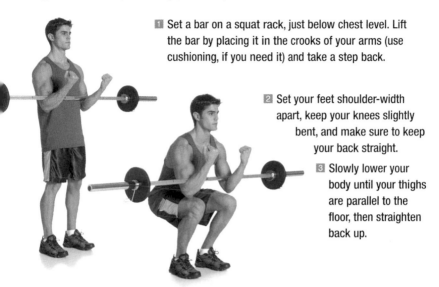

1 Set a bar on a squat rack, just below chest level. Lift the bar by placing it in the crooks of your arms (use cushioning, if you need it) and take a step back.

2 Set your feet shoulder-width apart, keep your knees slightly bent, and make sure to keep your back straight.

3 Slowly lower your body until your thighs are parallel to the floor, then straighten back up.

SQUAT VARIANT
OVERHEAD BAR SQUAT
Targets: Gluteals, Quadriceps, Hamstrings, Lower Back, Shoulders

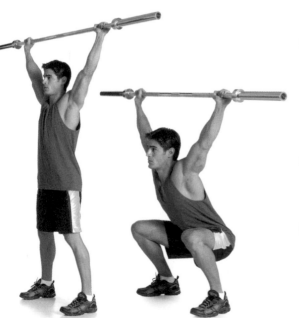

1 Standing with your feet shoulder-width apart, hold a barbell with an overhand grip. Press it over your head so your arms are fully extended.

2 Slowly lower your body, keeping your back in its natural alignment.

3 When your thighs are parallel to the floor, pause, then return to the starting position.

SQUAT VARIANT
HACK SQUAT
Targets: Quadriceps, Gluteals, Hamstrings

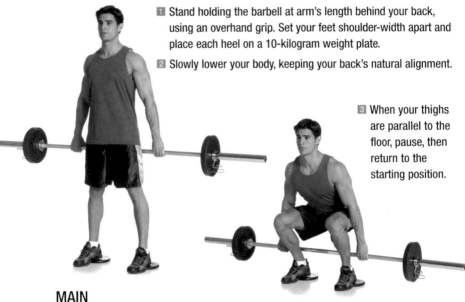

1 Stand holding the barbell at arm's length behind your back, using an overhand grip. Set your feet shoulder-width apart and place each heel on a 10-kilogram weight plate.

2 Slowly lower your body, keeping your back's natural alignment.

3 When your thighs are parallel to the floor, pause, then return to the starting position.

MAIN
BARBELL DEADLIFT
Targets: Gluteals, Hamstrings, Lower Back, Trapezius, Quadriceps

1 Squat in front of a barbell with your feet shoulder-width apart. Grab the barbell with an overhand grip, with your hands slightly wider than shoulder width. Keep your back straight or slightly arched. Keep your arms straight.

2 As you stand up, push down with your heels and pull the weight of the barbell to your body. Pause, then slowly return to the starting position. Repeat.

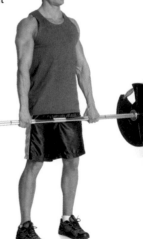

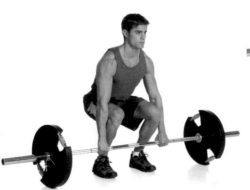

DEADLIFT VARIANT
KING DEADLIFT
Targets: Hamstrings, Gluteals, Lower Back

1 This exercise is done without weights. Stand with your knees slightly bent and your feet shoulder-width apart. Lift your right foot behind you and bend the knee 90 degrees so your right lower leg is almost parallel to the floor.

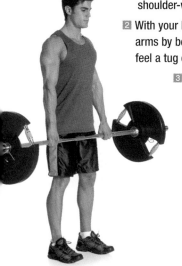

2 Slowly bend forwards at the hips until your left thigh is nearly parallel to the floor. Your right leg will rise as a counterbalance.

3 Pause, then bring your body back to the starting position.

TRAINER'S TIP
Do all the reps with one leg before switching to the other.

DEADLIFT VARIANT
ROMANIAN DEADLIFT
Targets: Hamstrings, Gluteals, Lower Back

1 Holding the barbell with an overhand grip, stand with your feet shoulder-width apart.

2 With your knees slightly bent, lower the barbell with straight arms by bending at the hips (keep your back straight) until you feel a tug or tension in your hamstrings.

3 Slowly return to the starting position.

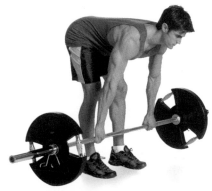

MAIN
BARBELL LUNGE
Targets: Quadriceps, Gluteals, Hamstrings

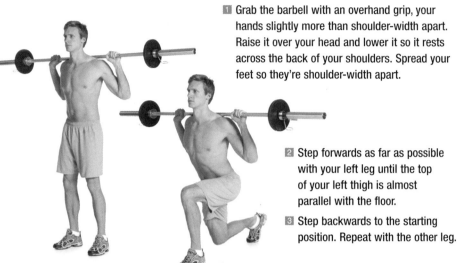

1. Grab the barbell with an overhand grip, your hands slightly more than shoulder-width apart. Raise it over your head and lower it so it rests across the back of your shoulders. Spread your feet so they're shoulder-width apart.

2. Step forwards as far as possible with your left leg until the top of your left thigh is almost parallel with the floor.

3. Step backwards to the starting position. Repeat with the other leg.

LUNGE VARIANT
45-DEGREE TRAVELLING LUNGE
Targets: Quadriceps, Gluteals, Hamstrings

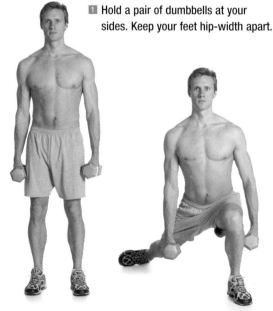

1. Hold a pair of dumbbells at your sides. Keep your feet hip-width apart.

2. Step forwards with your left leg and lower your body until your right knee almost touches the floor and your left knee is bent 90 degrees.

3. Stand and bring your right foot up next to your left. Repeat, with the right leg lunging forwards. That's 1 repetition.

Just a Few More

Now you know the 15 best exercises and you also have some variations to try. Here's a selection of great exercises that almost made the cut. Think of these as the runners-up.

LATERAL RAISE

Targets: Deltoids

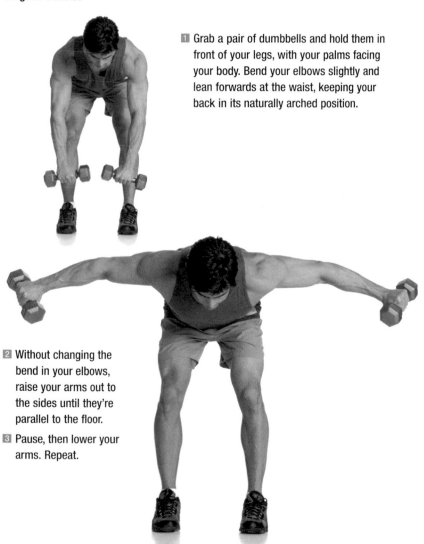

1 Grab a pair of dumbbells and hold them in front of your legs, with your palms facing your body. Bend your elbows slightly and lean forwards at the waist, keeping your back in its naturally arched position.

2 Without changing the bend in your elbows, raise your arms out to the sides until they're parallel to the floor.

3 Pause, then lower your arms. Repeat.

LEG PRESS
Targets: Quadriceps

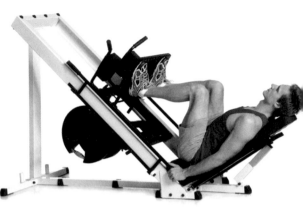

1 In the leg press station, sit with your back against the pad and your feet on the footplate, about shoulder-width apart. Your knees should be bent at slightly more than 90 degrees – adjust the seat if necessary.

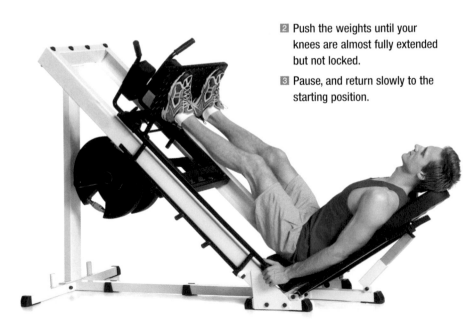

2 Push the weights until your knees are almost fully extended but not locked.

3 Pause, and return slowly to the starting position.

WIDE-GRIP LAT PULL-DOWN

Targets: Latissimus Dorsi, Trapezius, Biceps

1 Sit on the bench with your head and back straight. Grab the bar overhead with a wide, overhand grip (palms facing away from you).

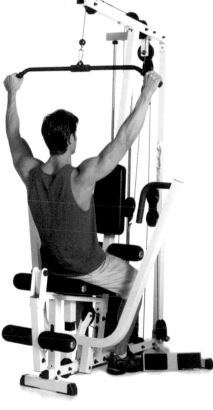

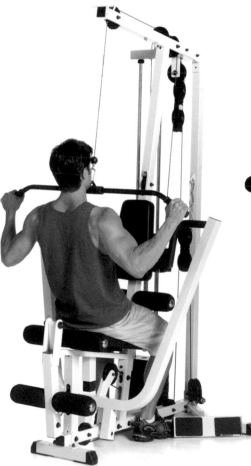

2 Moving only your arms, slowly pull the bar down towards your chest, squeezing your shoulder blades together while you pull down.

3 Pause, then slowly return to the starting position, resisting the weight as the bar rises.

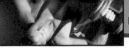

LYING LEG CURL
Targets: Hamstrings

1 Lie face down on a leg curl bench, with your knees hanging off the end. The bottom of your calves, just above the Achilles tendon, should hit the underside of the ankle pads.

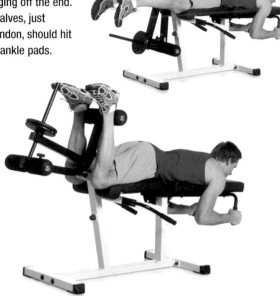

2 Bend your knees, lifting your lower legs up as far as they will go without touching your buttocks.

3 Pause, then slowly lower your legs until they are nearly straight.

MODIFIED FARMER'S WALK
Targets: Calves

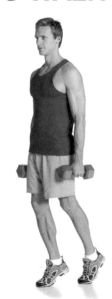

1 Grab a pair of heavy dumbbells and stand holding them at arm's length at your sides.

2 Stand on the balls of your feet and walk forwards until your grip is about to give out.

3 Put the dumbbells down, rest, then turn around and repeat, going back to the starting point.

TRAINER'S TIP
Don't let your heels touch the ground, or you won't get the full benefit of this exercise.

DUMBBELL CALF JUMP

Targets: Calves

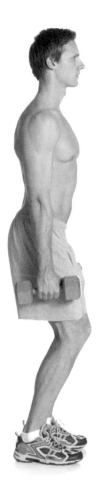

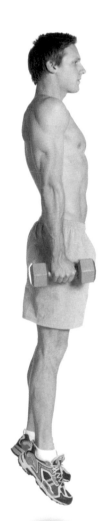

1 Stand with your feet hip-width apart. Grab a pair of dumbbells and hold them at your sides in a neutral grip at arm's length.

2 Dip your knees so they're bent about 45 degrees, then jump as high as you can. Point your toes towards the floor when you jump.

3 Allow your knees to bend 45 degrees when you land and then immediately jump again.

TRAINER'S TIP

Use much lighter dumbbells with this move – a little goes a long way. Use a quarter to a third of what you'd use for a Squat.

MAIN
SWISS BALL HIP EXTENSION AND LEG CURL

Targets: Lower Back, Abdominals, Gluteals, Hamstrings, Calves

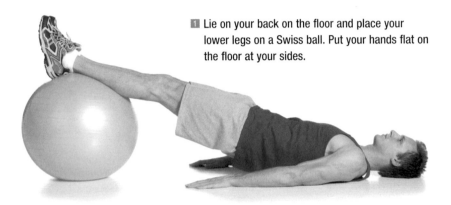

1 Lie on your back on the floor and place your lower legs on a Swiss ball. Put your hands flat on the floor at your sides.

2 Push your hips up so that your body forms a straight line from your shoulders to your ankles.

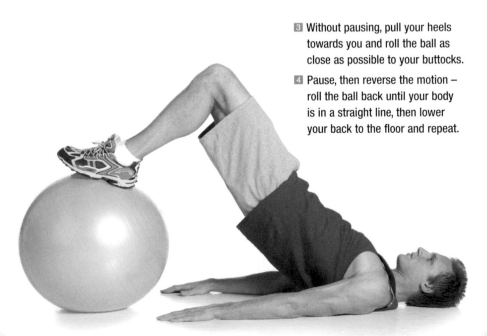

3 Without pausing, pull your heels towards you and roll the ball as close as possible to your buttocks.

4 Pause, then reverse the motion – roll the ball back until your body is in a straight line, then lower your back to the floor and repeat.

PART III:
Ultimate Workouts

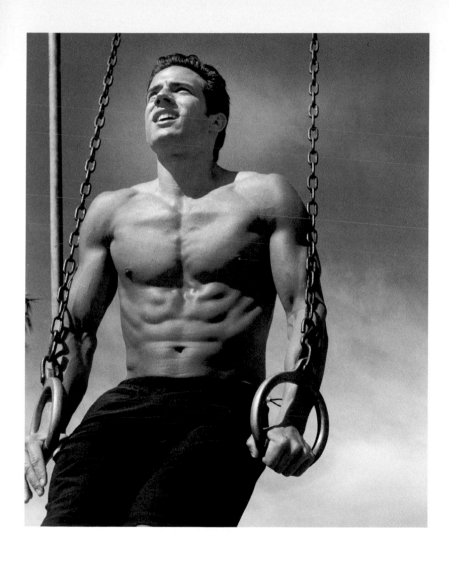

THE 15-MINUTE WORKOUT

Hard and Fast

This routine works all your major muscles in minimal time and burns fat by cranking up your metabolism. Do this workout three days a week, resting at least a day in between. Warm up with the first move using 60 per cent of the weight you can lift eight times. Then do two sets of eight reps with a weight you can lift 10 times with perfect form, resting one minute between sets.

Do the second and third exercises as a superset (one after the other, with no rest between). Perform eight reps of each with a weight you can lift with perfect form, and rest 45 seconds after each superset. Repeat each superset twice, using lighter weights for each set.

SUMO DEADLIFT

Targets: Quadriceps, Gluteals, Hamstrings, Lower Back, Trapezius, Adductors
Time: 5 minutes

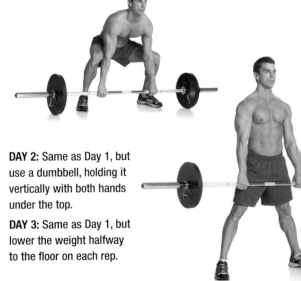

DAY 1: With your feet wider than shoulder width and your toes pointed out at about 45 degrees, grab the bar overhand with your hands inside your knees, shoulders over the bar, arms and back straight. Push down with your heels and stand up, keeping the bar in contact with your body. Finish standing upright with your shoulder blades back and down and your lower back flat. Pause, then lower the weight back to the floor.

DAY 2: Same as Day 1, but use a dumbbell, holding it vertically with both hands under the top.

DAY 3: Same as Day 1, but lower the weight halfway to the floor on each rep.

BARBELL BENCH PRESS

Targets: Pectorals, Front Deltoids, Triceps
Time: 5 minutes

DAY 1: Lie on a flat bench, holding the barbell over your chest with an overhand grip and straight arms. Lower the barbell until it just reaches your chest. Pause, then press the barbell back up.

DAY 2: Same as Day 1, but use 10 per cent less weight and lie on an incline bench.

DAY 3: Same as Day 1, but use 25 per cent less weight.

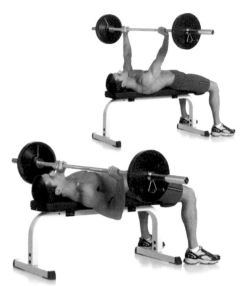

DUMBBELL BENT-OVER ROW

Targets: Upper and Mid-Back, Biceps
Time: 5 minutes

DAY 1: Hold a pair of dumbbells with an underhand grip and stand with your knees slightly bent. Bend at the hips and keep your lower back slightly arched. Pull the weights up until they're even with your lower ribcage. Pause, then return to the starting position.

DAY 2: Same as Day 1, but use an overhand grip and sit on an incline bench so your chest is against the pad. Keep your elbows flared out as you perform the row.

DAY 3: Same as Day 1, but use a neutral grip and bend forwards only about 30 degrees.

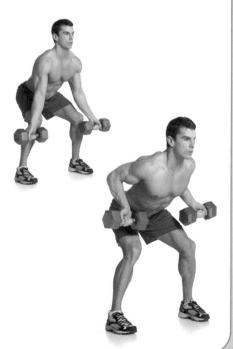

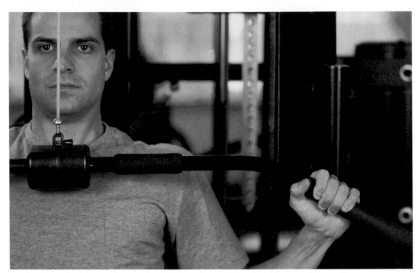

Staying focused on your workout, and not getting distracted by what others are doing, will help to establish a solid foundation at the gym.

Build Yourself a New Body

If you've reached the point where you would rather clean your toilet than look at your flabby self in the bathroom mirror, then it's time to build yourself a new body. The first four weeks of this total-body workout will increase strength and add definition. And if you keep it up for a few months, you'll find a new you smiling back from that mirror.

Benefits: How well you handle fatigue is often the difference between winning and losing a football match. It can make or break a workout programme, too. This routine teaches your muscles to continue working despite fatigue. It'll leave you feeling fresher in the second half and stronger in the final sets of your subsequent workouts.

Who's it for? A serious athlete or gym rat who wants to be able to perform better later in the game or near the end of a workout.

Beginner

Pace: Do the exercises with control three times a week, in the order listed.

Progress: Start with weights you can lift with perfect form 12 to 15 times. Increase weights each week, but only in amounts that allow you to maintain perfect form.

Rest: 1 minute between exercises.

Duration: Use this programme for 4 to 8 weeks if you are new to lifting or 2 to 3 weeks if you are coming back after some time away from the gym. When you can't increase the weight from one week to the next, you've peaked and are ready for the Advanced Beginner workout.

Advanced Beginner

Pace: Do the eight Advanced Beginner exercises three times a week as a total-body workout. After 3 to 4 weeks, substitute the exercises from the Beginner programme, but do them with the suggested Advanced Beginner sets and reps.

Progress: Increase weights with each set and every week.

Rest: 2 minutes between sets.

Duration: When you no longer find your strength and muscle size increasing or when you have the time and energy to do more exercises, you should switch to a more aggressive programme.

HITTING THE GYM FOR THE FIRST TIME

If you're a first-time lifter, you'll have a better chance of sticking with your workout if you take this advice. First, join a gym: there's a greater chance you'll create a routine if you work out somewhere other than home. Next, get some instruction: if your gym offers new members time with a trainer to learn the equipment and help with lifting form, take advantage of every minute. If your gym doesn't offer training, hire someone to instruct you for your first couple of workouts. The investment will pay off, as instruction will give you a foundation to refer to for every future workout. And lastly, find a partner: it may complicate your schedule, but you're less likely to skip a workout if someone (besides your girlfriend) is counting on you.

And, remember: don't change your workout every time you read a new bodybuilding article or see someone doing something interesting at the machine next to you. Add a multivitamin if you don't already take one, but otherwise just make sure you're eating fruits, vegetables, whole grains, low-fat dairy products and high-quality protein (eggs, fish, lean meat).

BEGINNER	
WEEKS 1–8	
EXERCISES	**REPS**
Leg press (p.66)	12–15
Lying leg curl (p.68)	12–15
Press-up (p.32)	12–15
Wide-grip lat pull-down (p.67)	12–15
Lying triceps extension (p.38)	12–15
Curl (p.34)	12–15
Triceps push-down (p.36)	12–15
Reverse crunch (p.56)	15–20
Superman (p.52)	15–20
Shoulder press (p.39)*	12–15
Cable upright row (p.46)*	12–15

*Add these exercises after the first week if you feel like doing more. But, if doing the nine sets in the workout above feels like enough of a workout for you, don't worry about these.

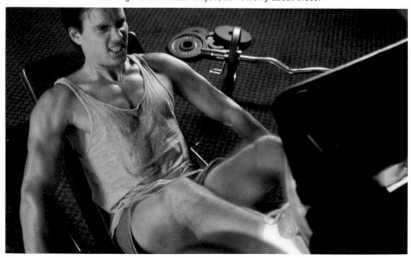

Leg presses help to build a powerful lower body, but use the position most comfortable for your knees.

ADVANCED BEGINNER

WEEKS 1–4

EXERCISES	SETS	REPS
Dumbbell squat (p.60)	3	12, 10, 8
Fly (p.47)	3	12, 10, 8
Cable row (p.45)	3	12, 10, 8
Seated barbell shoulder press (p.40)	3	12, 10, 8
Standing dumbbell biceps curl (p.35)	3	12, 10, 8
French press (p.41)	3	12, 10, 8
Crunch (p.55)	3	12, 10, 8
Back extension (p.51)	3	12, 10, 8

WEEKS 5–8

EXERCISES	SETS	REPS
Leg press (p.66)	3	12, 10, 8
Lying leg curl (p.68)	3	12, 10, 8
Barbell bench press (p.39)	3	12, 10, 8
Wide-grip lat pull-down (p.67)	3	12, 10, 8
Lying triceps extension (p.38)	3	12, 10, 8
Curl (p.34)	3	12, 10, 8
Triceps push-down (p.36)	3	12, 10, 8
Reverse crunch (p.56)	3	12, 10, 8
Superman (p.52)	3	12, 10, 8
Shoulder press (p.39)*	3	12, 10, 8
Cable upright row (p.46)*	3	12, 10, 8

*Add these exercises if you feel ready and have energy left after completing the other exercises.

THE 15-MINUTE WORKOUT

Count Down to Build Up Fast

Try this descending-repetition workout, with little rest between sets. Short rest periods stimulate the release of growth hormone, which builds muscle and burns fat. Alternate the workouts: in the first week, perform Workout A on Monday and Friday, and Workout B on Wednesday. Flip that in the second week. Use 50 to 60 per cent of the weight you can lift once. Do 10 repetitions, rest 10 seconds without letting go of the bar, then nine reps, rest 10 seconds, eight reps, and so on, down to one. (For Pull-ups, start with five.) Rest two minutes between exercises.

Benefits: It's a quick but tough total-body workout. It'll leave you looking forward to your next workout.

Who's it for? It's intended for intermediate to advanced lifters who have more skill than time.

Quick workouts keep your muscles warm; short rests between sets helps to build muscle while burning fat.

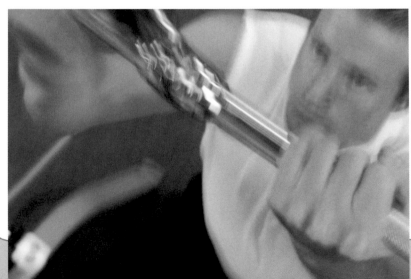

Workout A

BARBELL SQUAT

Targets: Gluteals, Quadriceps, Hamstrings, Lower Back
Time: 7.5 minutes

1 Set a barbell on a squat rack and grab it with an overhand grip; step under the bar so it rests across your upper back. Lift it off the rack and step back, feet shoulder-width apart.

2 Lower your body, keeping your back in its natural alignment and your lower legs nearly perpendicular to the floor. When your thighs are parallel to the floor or lower, pause, then return to the starting position.

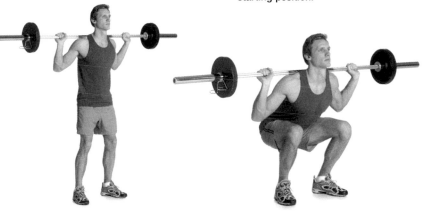

BARBELL BENCH PRESS

Targets: Pectorals, Front Deltoids, Triceps
Time: 7.5 minutes

1 Grab the bar with your hands just wider than shoulder width and hold it over your chest at arm's length.

2 Lower the bar to your chest, pause, then push it straight up to the starting position.

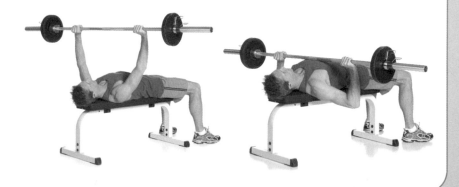

Workout B

BARBELL DEADLIFT

Targets: Gluteals, Hamstrings, Lower Back, Trapezius, Quadriceps
Time: 7.5 minutes

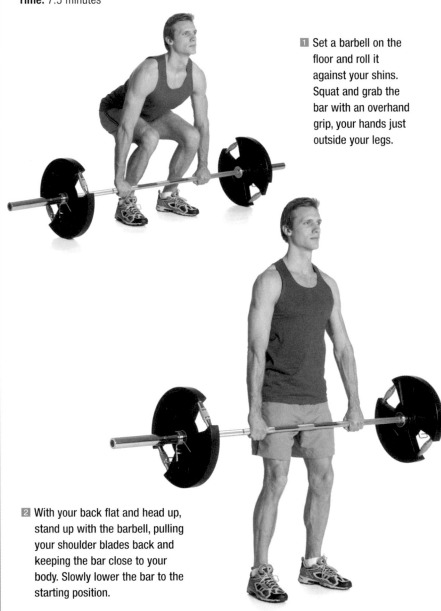

■ Set a barbell on the floor and roll it against your shins. Squat and grab the bar with an overhand grip, your hands just outside your legs.

② With your back flat and head up, stand up with the barbell, pulling your shoulder blades back and keeping the bar close to your body. Slowly lower the bar to the starting position.

UNDERHAND PULL-UP

Targets: Upper and Mid-Back, Biceps
Time: 7.5 minutes

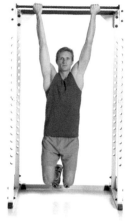

1 Grab a pull-up bar with a shoulder-width, underhand grip. Hang at arm's length.

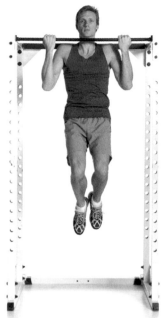

2 Pull yourself up as high as you can. Pause, then slowly return to the starting position.

SUPERSETS FOR STRENGTH AND POWER

Most of us use the words 'strength' and 'power' interchangeably, but they're actually two different qualities. Strength is measured by the amount of weight you can move, at any speed. Power is weight times speed, or the ability to knock an inanimate object into the next time zone. The strength/power combo enables you to work with heavier weights, so you build muscle faster.

Try a five-repetition set of a heavy-duty strength exercise, like the Squat shown on page 60. Then, do 5 to 10 repetitions of a power exercise – one that involves moving your body as fast as possible while holding a lighter load. Try doing a Dumbbell Calf Jump (page 69) as the second exercise of this superset. Stand holding a pair of dumbbells at arm's length at your sides. Squat down about halfway, then immediately jump as high as you can. Bend your knees as you land. Regain your balance, then repeat.

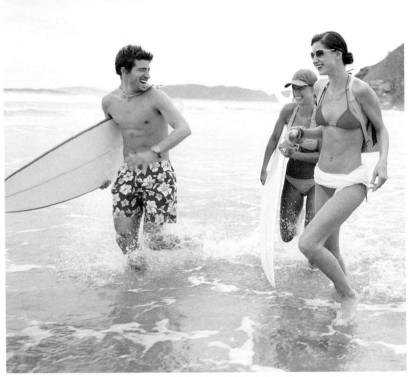

When it's time to leave your shirt behind, you'll thank yourself for staying with your workout.

Beach-Ready Body in 4 Weeks

A little time spent on the proper workout can transform your body and make it a summer to remember on the beach. You can do the exercises at your gym exactly as they are listed here, or do barbell or dumbbell versions at the gym or at home. Or, you can splurge and buy a multistation home gym so you can do the gym versions without having to leave home.

BEGINNER WORKOUT A: UPPER BODY

	EXERCISES	REPS
Complex 1	Shoulder press (p.39)	8, 10, 12
	Piston upright row (p.47)	8, 10, 12
	Lateral raise (p.65)	8, 10, 12
Complex 2	Bench dip (p.43)	8, 10, 12
	Lying triceps extension (p.38)	8, 10, 12
	Wide-grip lat pull-down (p.67)	8, 10, 12
	Cable biceps curl (p.35)	8, 10, 12

BEGINNER WORKOUT B: LOWER BODY

	EXERCISES	REPS
Complex 1	Front squat (p.60)	8, 10, 12
	Situp (p.59)	8, 10, 12
Complex 2	King deadlift (p.63)	8, 10, 12
	Incline reverse crunch (p.57)	8, 10, 12
Complex 3	45-degree travelling lunge (p.64)	8, 10, 12
	V-Up (p.59)	8, 10, 12

Benefits: Not only do you build muscle mass, you also challenge your muscles' endurance by performing multiple exercises for the same muscles without taking a break in between.

Who's it for? The guy who wants to build muscle fast. It also burns off as much fat as possible by using the biggest muscles to crank up the metabolism. Ideally, this total-body workout is designed to help you feel good about taking your shirt off, whether in the bedroom or at the beach.

Who's Who

Do the Beginner workout if you've been doing strength training for less than a year or if you are starting

INTERMEDIATE/ADVANCED WORKOUT A: UPPER BODY

EXERCISES	REPS
Complex 1 Shoulder press (p.39)	6, 8, 10
Piston upright row (p.47)	6, 8, 10
Lateral raise (p.65)	6, 8, 10
Complex 2 Weighted dip (p.44)	6, 8, 10
Lying triceps extension (p.38)	6, 8, 10
Close-grip overhand pull-up (p.88)	6, 8, 10
Cable biceps curl (p.35)	6, 8, 10

INTERMEDIATE/ADVANCED WORKOUT B: LOWER BODY

EXERCISES	REPS
Complex 1 Front squat (p.60)	6, 8, 10
Situp (p. 59)	6, 8, 10
Complex 2 King deadlift (p.63)	6, 8, 10
Swiss ball jackknife (p.58)	6, 8, 10
Complex 3 45-degree travelling lunge (p.64)	6, 8, 10
V-up (p.59)	6, 8, 10

back after a layoff of four months or longer. If you've worked out regularly for the past year, do the Intermediate/Advanced programme.

Frequency

For the Beginner and Intermediate/Advanced programmes, do Workout A (Upper Body) twice a week and Workout B (Lower Body) once a week, resting one day after each workout. For example, do Workout A on Monday and Friday and Workout B on Wednesday.

Pace

In each workout, perform each complex of exercises as a circuit, doing one exercise after another with no

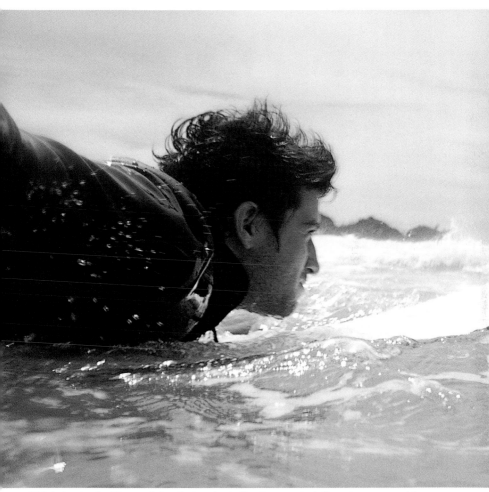

Well-designed and solidly-executed workouts on land will make your swim to the surf seem even quicker. And who knows? It might even help you to stay on the board just a little longer.

rest in between. After you've completed one circuit, rest 90 seconds, and then repeat the complex twice more for a total of three sets of each exercise. Rest 90 seconds, and then begin the exercises in the next complex. For each complex, use a reverse pyramid system: start with heavy weights and a low number of repetitions for your first set, then reduce the weight and increase the reps for each subsequent set.

Beginners should do eight repetitions in the first set of exercises, 10 in the second and 12 in the third. Intermediate/Advanced lifters should do six reps in the first set of exercises, eight in the second and 10 in the third.

Supersets: More Muscle in Less Time

Supersets are the extra-value meals of exercise: more of what you want, at a lower cost. They can give you more muscle in less time, with less energy expenditure and even less boredom. Here's the basic idea behind supersets: you alternate between sets of different exercises with little rest in between, rather than knock out all your sets of one exercise before moving on to the next. For example, a workout that normally takes 24 minutes could be cut to 20. And because you take more time between sets of an exercise, you can use more weight when you lift – more muscle, less time.

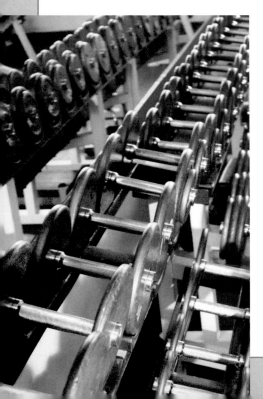

Supersets for Bigger Muscles

Your muscles have two types of fibres. The smaller, slow-twitch fibres are used primarily for endurance activities, and the bigger, fast-twitch fibres mostly come into play when you need to move a heavy object, or move a light object fast. Work them all if you want the biggest muscles possible. Do 10 repetitions of one exercise, then 20 repetitions of a different exercise for the same muscle group, without rest. Then rest 60 seconds and repeat. Two or three of the following supersets is sufficient.

There are plenty of weights to choose from at most gyms. The key is not to do too much too fast and knowing when to increase the weights.

INCLINE DUMBBELL BENCH PRESS

Targets: Chest, Triceps, Front Shoulders
Reps: 10

1 Set an incline bench to about 30 degrees.

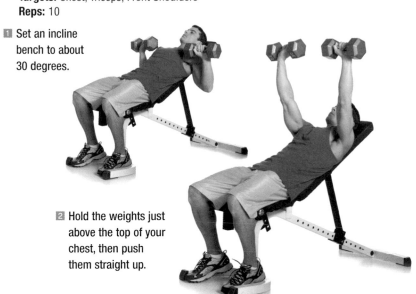

2 Hold the weights just above the top of your chest, then push them straight up.

PRESS-UP

Targets: Abdominals, Triceps, Pectorals
Reps: 20

1 Get on the floor with your back straight and your body weight resting on your palms and toes.

2 Lower yourself to the floor, then push back up.

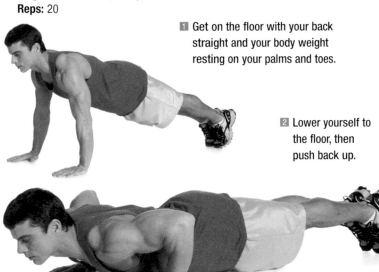

CLOSE-GRIP OVERHAND PULL-UP

Targets: Latissimus Dorsi, Biceps
Reps: 10

1 Grab a pull-up bar with an overhand grip, your hands 15 to 30 centimetres apart. Hang at arm's length.

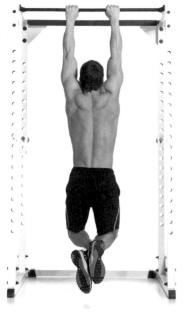

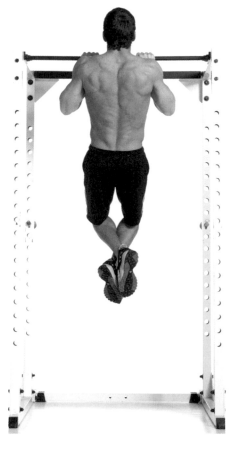

2 Now pull your chin up over the bar, pause, and lower yourself back down.

WIDE-GRIP LAT PULL-DOWN

Targets: Latissimus Dorsi, Trapezius, Biceps
Reps: 20

1 Grab the bar with the widest possible overhand grip.

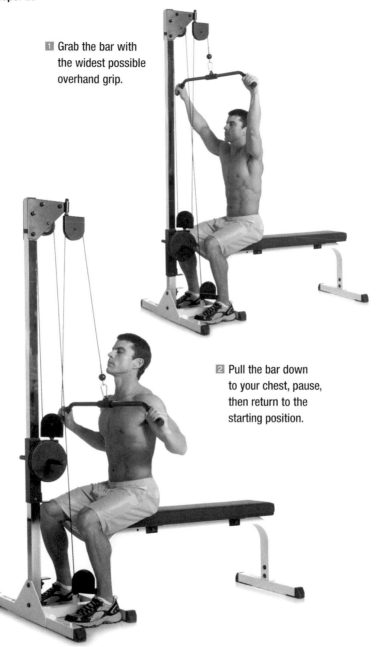

2 Pull the bar down to your chest, pause, then return to the starting position.

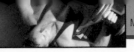

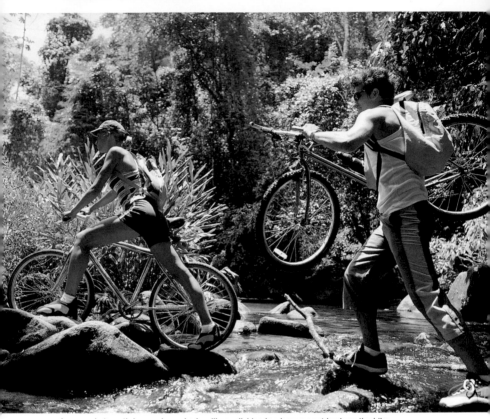

Increased strength in your lower body will pay dividends when you get back on the bike.

The Power of Your Lower Body

If you want your legs to catch the eye of every woman in the park or on the beach, this workout is for you. The exercises included here force your muscles to work the way they would while playing sport and doing other outdoor activities. The extra intensity in the lower-body workout (plus the upper-body exercises) will build extra muscle that is sure to get you noticed.

REACHING YOUR TOP FORM

You can use this workout as a total-body programme by doing a series of upper-body lifts after you've done the leg and buttocks exercises. You can do the lower body portion of the exercises in any order, but try to increase the weight you lift in each exercise by 5 to 10 per cent each week. Instructions on how to transform each of these workouts into total-body programmes (for Beginner, Intermediate and Advanced) are included on pages 92–94. Make sure you include extra time to work your whole body. It's time well spent.

And, remember: it's important that you work out with equal effort on both sides as well as the front and back of your body. Concentrating just on your dominant side or the front (because it's what you see in the mirror) is asking for trouble in the form of injury. You ignore any body part at your own peril.

Benefits: The best way to build new muscle mass is to find a new way to work your muscles, and this workout provides the exercises and techniques to do just that.

Who's it for? This is a creative workout routine for the guy who's willing to learn some new exercises and at the same time challenge his muscles in different ways.

Who's Who

If you are new to weight training or have taken a long break from it, you're classified as a beginner. You're considered an intermediate if you've been lifting from six months to a year, have tried several different workout programmes, and have seen gains in strength and muscle mass. You've graduated to advanced lifter status if you've been training regularly for more than a year, you've made considerable gains in strength and size, you're proficient in squats and several varieties of deadlifts and you can do at least five pull-ups.

Frequency

Do the lower body exercises for your experience level for four weeks, two sets the first two weeks and two or three sets during the last two weeks. Advanced lifters should do this workout after a thorough warmup with lighter weights.

Lifters, especially at the Beginner and Intermediate level, must ensure that they warm up properly before a workout. Five to 10 minutes of aerobic exercise at a comfortable pace – jogging or skipping – is a good start. To prevent muscle soreness, do a similar cool-down when you're done.

BEGINNER		
EXERCISES **LOWER-BODY ROUTINE**	**WEEKS 1–2** REPS	**WEEKS 3–4** REPS
Modified farmer's walk (p.68)	10–12	8–10
45-degree travelling lunge (p.64)	10–12	8–10
King deadlift (p.63)	10–12	8–10
Swiss ball hip extension and leg curl (p.70)	10–12	8–10
Front squat (p.60)	10–12	8–10
UPPER-BODY ROUTINE		
Wide-grip lat pull-down (p.67)	8–12	8–12
Barbell bench press (p.39)	8–12	8–12
Cable upright row (p.46)	8–12	8–12
Triceps push-down (p.36)	8–12	8–12
Standing dumbbell biceps curl (p.35)	8–12	8–12
Crunch (p.55)	15–20	15–20

Beginner

Do a total-body workout all in one session two or three times a week. After doing the lower-body exercises, try one set of 8 to 12 repetitions of the upper-body routine. This is an ideal start to a better body.

Intermediate

Divide your training into two workouts, one for upper body and one for lower body. Alternate between the two, with a day of rest after each workout. For example, if you do the lower-body workout from the chart on Monday and Friday, do an upper-body workout on Wednesday. The next week, do the opposite.

You should also do some abdominal exercises on the day you work out your lower body. That will ensure that you are working your entire body, avoiding the workout pitfall of focusing on one area.

Your upper-body workout should be made up of one exercise each, of

INTERMEDIATE		
EXERCISES	**WEEKS 1–2**	**WEEKS 3–4**
LOWER-BODY ROUTINE, PLUS ABS	**REPS**	**REPS**
Overhead bar squat (p.61)	8–10	6–8
Hack squat (p.62)	8–10	6–8
Swiss ball hip extension and leg curl (p.70)	8–10	6–8
Dumbbell calf jump (p.69)	8–10	6–8
Single-leg back extension (p.52)	8–10	6–8
Crunch (p.55)	15–20	15–20
V-Up (p.59)	15–20	15–20
UPPER-BODY ROUTINE		
Cable row OR Barbell bent-over row (p.45)	8–12	8–12
Barbell bench press (p.39)	8–12	8–12
Overhand pull-up (p.48) OR Wide-grip lat pull-down (p.67)	8–12	8–12
Shoulder press (p.39)	8–12	8–12
Lying triceps extension (p.38)	8–12	8–12
Standing dumbbell biceps curl (p.35)	8–12	8–12

horizontal pulling (Cable Row or Barbell Bent-Over Row), horizontal pushing (Barbell Bench Press), vertical pulling (Overhand Pull-up or Wide-Grip Lat Pull-down) and vertical pushing (Barbell Shoulder Press).

Some tips that will help to maximize your time while at the gym:

1. Lift the weights as fast possible. This allows you to use heavier weights and boost your total.
2. Lower the weights slowly – take perhaps four seconds to maximize benefits.
3. Rest a minute or less between sets – keep the pace going.

Advanced

Divide your workout into three parts: vertical push and pull, lower-body exercises plus abdominals, and horizontal push and pull. Do each workout once a week and take a day off in between. Your body will appreciate the effort.

ADVANCED		
EXERCISES **VERTICAL PUSH AND PULL**	**WEEKS 1–2** REPS	**WEEKS 3–4** REPS
Shoulder press (p.39)	8–12	8–12
Overhand pull-up (p.48) OR Wide-grip lat pull-down (p.67)	8–12	8–12
LOWER BODY ROUTINE, PLUS ABS		
Overhead bar squat (p.61)	6–8	4–6
Hack squat (p.62)	6–8	4–6
Swiss ball hip extension and leg curl (p.70)	6–8	4–6
Dumbbell calf jump (p.69)	6–8	4–6
Single-leg back extension (p.52)	6–8	4–6
Crunch (p.55)	15–20	15–20
Hanging knee raise (p.53)	15–20	15–20
HORIZONTAL PUSH AND PULL	**REPS**	**REPS**
Cable row OR Barbell bent-over row (p.45)	8–12	8–12
Barbell bench press (p.39)	8–12	8–12

INDEX